J.-F. GINESTIE and A. ROMIEU

Radiologist,
Montpellier

Sexologist,
Montpellier

W0050695

radiologic exploration of impotence

With 80 Roentgenograms

MARTINUS NIJHOFF MEDICAL DIVISION
THE HAGUE / BOSTON / LONDON

1978

ISBN-13: 978-90-247-2023-1   e-ISBN-13: 978-94-009-9683-0
DOI: 10.1007/978-94-009-9683-0

Softcover reprint of the hardcover 1st edition 1978

radiologic
exploration
of impotence

Acknowledgments

We wish to thank

Doctor Andrée GINESTIE, who helped us in our explorations and made the diagrams of this book ;

Doctor Jean GINESTIE, our coworker, who performs the microsurgical catheterizations of **arteriae dorsalis penis** *and the surgical interventions on our patients.*

CONTENTS

LIST OF ILLUSTRATIONS

ABBREVIATIONS

F :	Gluteal artery
0 :	Obturator artery
T I H :	Ischio-pudental trunk
H I :	Internal pudental artery
H I Ac :	Accessory internal pudental artery
P S :	Perineal superficial artery
B :	Artery of penial bulb
C :	Deep artery
D V :	Dorsal artery of penis
I :	Ischial artery
E :	Epigastric artery
Circ :	Circonflex circle

INTRODUCTION

Though impotence is a disease as old as man, it is very little known. For centuries sexual pathology was hidden behind a veil of shame and decency, and this accounts for our ignorance in this field. Freud was the first to impose upon us its existence. However, the somatically-oriented physician kept ignoring the diseases of this new chapter of pathology since they offered no approach to his knowledge and methods of diagnosis.

In sexual pathology, the disease of an individual is always associated with a problem of relationship with another person, a pathologic state of the « other », acting as cause, factor or consequence of the disturbance awaiting diagnosis and treatment. It is no longer one person who has to be examined, but a couple.

Impotence, the subject of this book, can be a symptom or a disease. As a symptom, it may occur in certain symptom complexes such as Leriche's syndrome. As a disease, it is the only manifestation or disturbance that worries the patient and of which he wants to be cured.

Erection can be defined as dilation and hardening of the erectile organs, thus the cavernous and spongy bodies. It is a vascular phenomenon (turgescence of vascular spaces) under neurologic control. Impotence is the lack or insufficiency of erection.

This monograph purports to study rœntgenologically the vascular organs which are necessary to achieve erection, and their pathologic modifications causing impotence. The findings are based on our experience with 250 patients whose examinations included 460 arteriograms of the internal iliac artery and 52 rœntgenograms of the cavernous bodies. The explored vascular organs were arteries, erectile tissues and veins of drainage.

The first part of the book deals with the studies of arteries : techniques of exploration, normal and pathologic rœntgenograms. We will not discuss the large vessels, i.e. the abdominal aorta and the common and external iliac arteries, since their pathology is well-known. When these arteries are the cause of impotence, the latter is only a symptom : the patient complains of pain in his lower limbs during walking or in recumbency. By contrast, there are more distally located lesions involving the internal pudendal arteries or the deep arteries of the penis, which cause only impotence and which have until now not as yet been studied. To present this neglected chapter of pathology is the particular purpose of this publication.

The second part deals with the study of the erectile organs. It is necessarily smaller since until now we have only found significant changes in Peyronie's disease.

There is no chapter on the veins of drainage since we have not observed any venous lesion in relation to impotence. Our explorations of veins are used only for our anatomic studies and our research in hemodynamics.

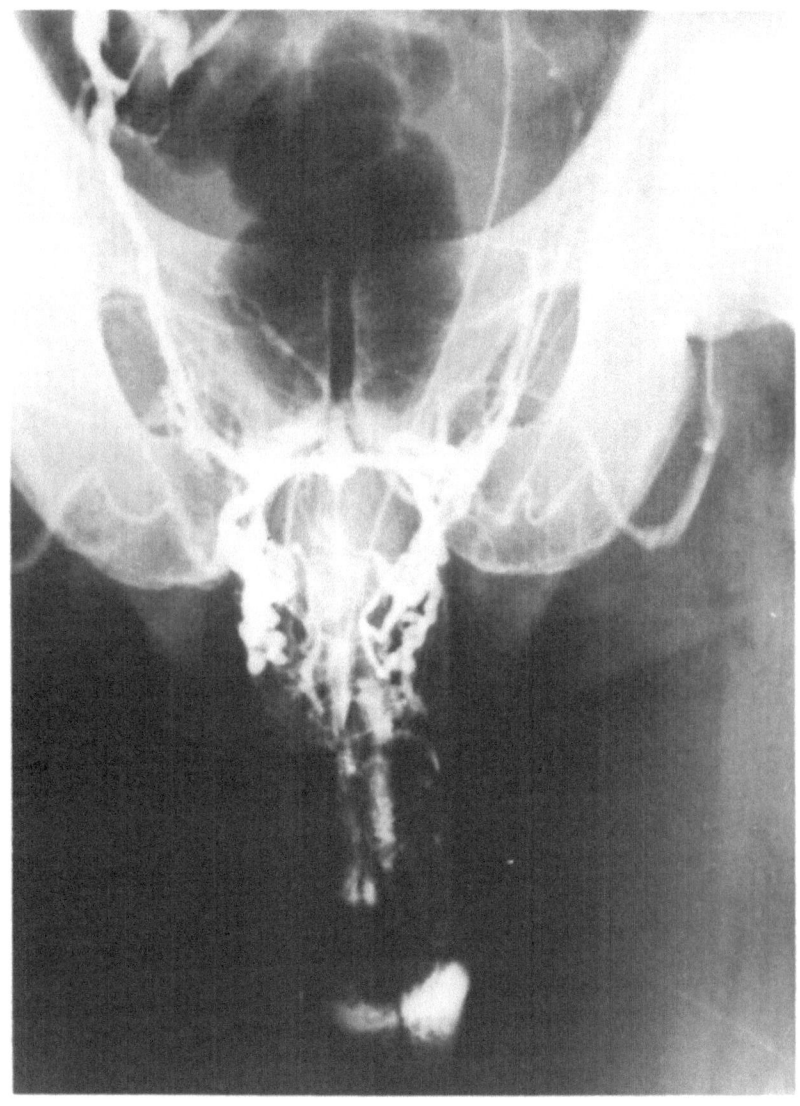

Fig. 1 - Retrograde phlebography of deep dorsal vein of penis

Corpus spongiosum is only opacified by this means.

There is no retrograde injection of corpus cavernosum.

This investigation permits a study of venous draining of erectile organs and a hemodynamic study.

ARTERIOGRAPHY OF INTERNAL PUDENDAL ARTERY

TECHNIQUES

I) ARTERIAL CATHETERIZATION

— Puncture of the axillary artery
— Puncture of the femoral artery
— Puncture of the dorsal artery of the penis
— Choice of approach

II) PROJECTIONS

— Basic projections
— Complementary projections

III) OPACIFICATION

IV) RECORDING

The arteriographic exploration is performed under anesthesia. The use of radiopaque substances in the internal iliac (hypogastric) arteries is more painful than in the limbs and would not be accepted by the patient. Certain substances, such as Palfium *, used during anesthesia, lead to better pictures.

I) ARTERIAL CATHETERIZATION

Radiopaque material can be introduced into the internal pudendal and penile arteries through the left axillary artery, the femoral arteries, or, if necessary, the dorsal arteries of the penis. Because of the small lumina of the vessels to be explored and the small amount of fluid that is necessary, the catheters used are likewise of small calibers (maximum caliber : red catheter of Odman). A very fine silicone catheter is required for the retrograde arteriography of the dorsal artery of the penis.

Puncture of the axillary artery

● Only the left axillary artery needs to be punctured and only one catheter needs to be introduced into the aorta. The tip of the catheter forms a wide open angle of 160 degrees. The exploration is performed in two or three stages :

1) The tip of the catheter is advanced to the subrenal portion of the abdominal aorta in order to study the aortic cross-roads.

---

* Dextromoramide.

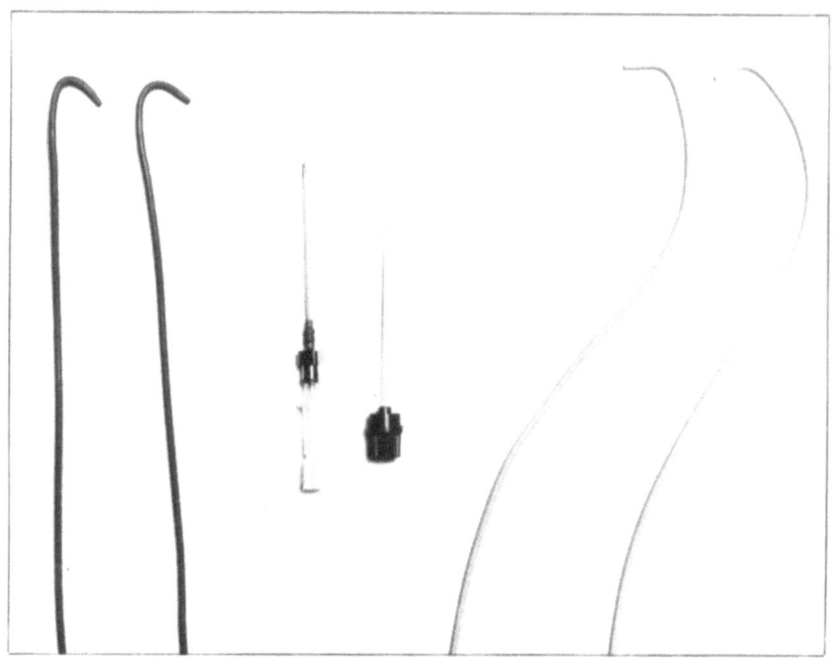

Fig. 2 - Materials used for hypogastric arteriographies

Trocars fo femoral artery punctures. Retrograde aortography may also be realized by this means.

Slightly curved catheters of small caliber for hypogastric artery catheterizations.

COBRA catheters for hyperselective arteriographies.

2) The catheter is directed selectively into the right internal iliac artery, then into the left one.

3) (Optional). The axillary approach allows in general an easy superselective catheterization of the right and left internal pudendal arteries.

● The advantages of this approach are : the need of only one arterial puncture and only one catheter for the entire procedure ; and the easiness of superselective arteriography.

● The disadvantages are those of any axillary arteriography : proximity of the brachial plexus ; difficulties in certain cases in the catheterization of the descending portion of the thoracic aorta ; and greater seriousness of thrombosis, should such accident occur.

Puncture of the femoral artery

● Both femoral arteries must be punctured. The tip of the catheter, bent at a very acute angle, must be small so that it may enter the iliac artery. Too long a tip would make it difficult or impossible to penetrate the internal iliac artery and would risk a dissection of the intima at the level of the origin of this vessel.

● As in the case of the axillary artery, the exploration proceeds in two or three stages :

1) The femoral arteries are entered by flexible silicone catheters which are less traumatizing and more easily manipulated than the usual metallic trocarts. The aortic crossroads are studied after retrograde bifemoral injection.

2) The catheters are positioned according to Seldinger's technique. The catheterization of the right and left internal iliac arteries presents no difficulty.

3) (Optional). The superselective catheterization of the internal pudendal arteries necessitates a change of catheter. It can be done :

— *with Cobra curve catheters :* in about two thirds of the cases, in spite of the very acute angle formed by the junction of the internal with the external iliac artery, these catheters facilitate superselective homolateral catheterization of the internal pudendal artery. In case this should be impossible, crosswise catheterization can be performed using the left femoral Cobra catheter for the right internal pudendal artery and the right femoral catheter for the left internal pudendal ;

— *with a double catheter :* the first catheter (black type Odman) enters the internal iliac artery. The second catheter, with very thin walls, is introduced into the lumen of the first one. The superselective catheterization of the internal pudendal artery is facilitated by a guide wire.

● The advantages of this approach are those of any femoral arteriography. If it is performed by a skilled operator there is almost never any accident or incident.

● The disadvantages are minor. Both femoral arteries must be punctured and superselective catheterization is less easy.

Puncture of the dorsal artery of the penis

● This is a surgical procedure. It consists of the denudation of the distal third of the artery and its retrograde catheterization by a very fine silicone catheter under microscopic control.

● By this approach the penile arteries (dorsal and deep arteries of the penis, artery of bulb of penis) are very well visualized. It is not possible to visualize the internal pudendal artery beyond the origin of the perineal artery.

● The advantages of this approach are the perfect visualization of the penile arteries and the possibility to study them in case of an obstacle upstream.

● The disadvantage is obvious. It is a microsurgical technique which requires the cooperation of a surgeon with specialized skill.

Choice of approach

● We prefer the femoral to the axillary approach, using the latter only in exceptional cases. We examine routinely the aortic crossroads, except in individuals under 35 years of age who have no vascular deficiency. We use superselective catheterization only rarely and always on second intention.

● In some cases, the penile arteries do not arise from the internal pudendal artery. An isolated superselective arteriography of the internal pudendal artery could give the false impression that they do not exist. The images obtained by superselective arteriography are not better than those obtained by internal iliac arteriography. In the case of an obstacle with poor collaterals, superselective arteriography rarely improves the visualization of the area downstream.

● A scratch of the intima in these arteries of very fine caliber and of very small blood flow could produce thrombosis and aggravate the syndrome of impotence.

● Retrograde arteriography of the dorsal artery of the penis is a complementary examination. We use it in two instances :

   — One or more penile arteries are not visualized by internal pudendal arteriography in a patient considered for a surgical intervention.

   — In a current research project on the hemodynamics of the erectile organs.

II) PROJECTIONS

Three basic views, used in every patient, permit precise arteriographic assessment of the lesions in.the majority of cases. In case of disturbing superpositions, doubtful or unprecise films, additional views are sometimes needed. Their choice depends upon the arterial segment presenting the problem.

A) BASIC PROJECTIONS

Frontal view

It is centered on the aortic crossroads and the iliac arteries and is used for the first part of the examination, infrarenal aortography.

Right and left oblique views

These are used for the study of the internal iliac, the internal pudendal, and the penile arteries.

● For the injection of the right axes, the patient's pelvis is placed in the right anterior oblique position. The penis is stabilized on the left thigh so as to receive the radiations laterally. A sack of four is placed on the penis in order to equalize the densities and to obtain an uniformly clear image of the internal iliac artery, the internal pudendal artery, and the penile arteries.

● For the injection of the left axes, the sides are reversed.

● These two oblique views do not necessitate catheterization of the bladder, since the involved arteries are seen completely outside and below the projection of the bladder. However, during the first examinations the presence of an indwelling catheter is useful. Its opacification by the contrast fluid eliminated with the urine makes the urethra visible on the films and allows for a better differentiation of the arteries leading to the penis from those going to the scrotum.

B) COMPLEMENTARY PROJECTIONS

In order to avoid the superposition of any bladder shadow, the bladder should be emptied by catheterization.

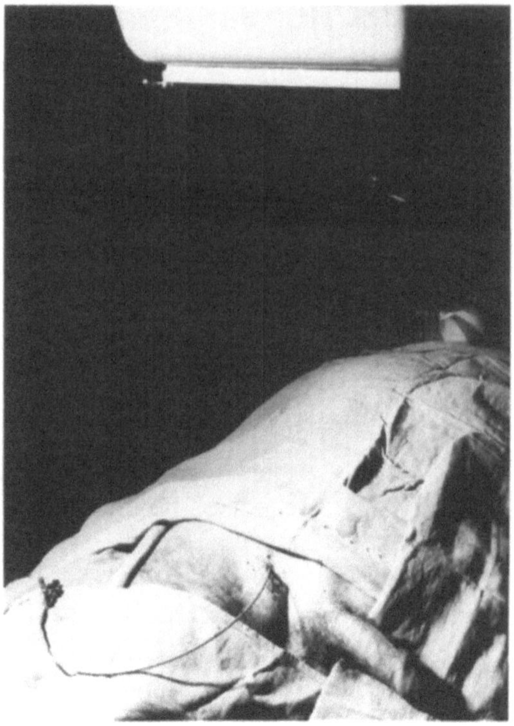

Fig. 3 - Internal pudental arteriography - projection

Patient placed in oblique postion.

Penis stabilized on opposite thigh to artery to be radiographed.

X ray beam positioned vertically towards artery.

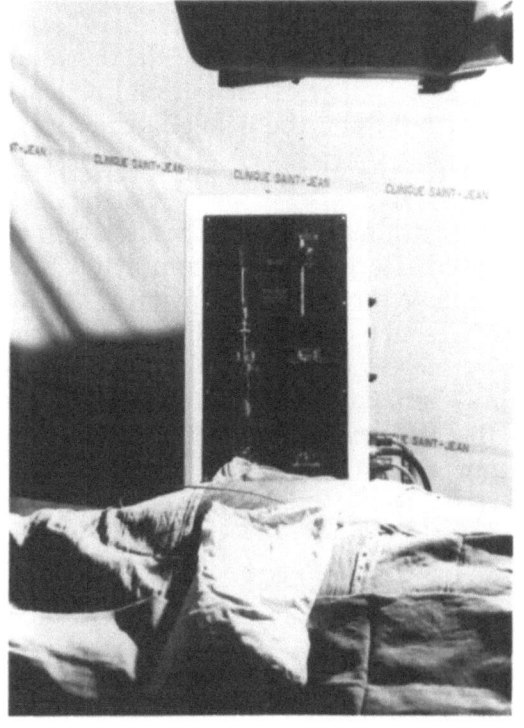

Fig. 4 - Internal pudendal arteriography - technique

It is essential to place a sack of flour on penis to equalize the densities and permit penial arteries to be seen.

Right and left oblique views

These may complement the front of view for the study of the terminal portion of the abdominal aorta and the iliac arteries. The left anterior oblique view during the opacification of the right axes and the right anterior oblique view during the opacification of the left axes complement the opposite obliques for the study of the internal iliac arteries and the abdominal and gluteal portions of the internal pudendal arteries.

Ascending oblique view

The patient is recumbent. His penis is reclined and stabilized on his abdomen in an exactly symmetric position. The rays are directed upward at an angle of between 25 and 30 degrees. This view is used for the study of the perineal portion of the internal pudendal arteries and for the penile arteries.

III) OPACIFICATION

The arteries to be visualized are of very small caliber and have a light blood flow. A hydrosoluble contrast fluid of the lowest possible degree of viscosity is necessary. We use preheated Télébrix 30. A good amount of fluid must be injected ; each internal iliac arteriography requires a volume of 60 ml. The injection must be done at slow speed, over a period of 20 seconds, i.e. 3 milliliters per second. A heavier flow would result in a reflux of the contrast fluid into the external iliac artery and in less good visualization.

IV) RECORDING

A serialograph is needed and the films must be 35 cm by 35 cm. The speed of exposure is slow : one film per second. Serialography starts 10 seconds after the beginning of the injection and continues over a period of 20 seconds.

Subtraction technique is exceptionally useful. Magnification films with a 0.1 focus would be of greatest usefulness for the study of the penile arteries, particularly the deep artery of the penis.

ARTERIOGRAPHY OF INTERNAL PUDENDAL ARTERY

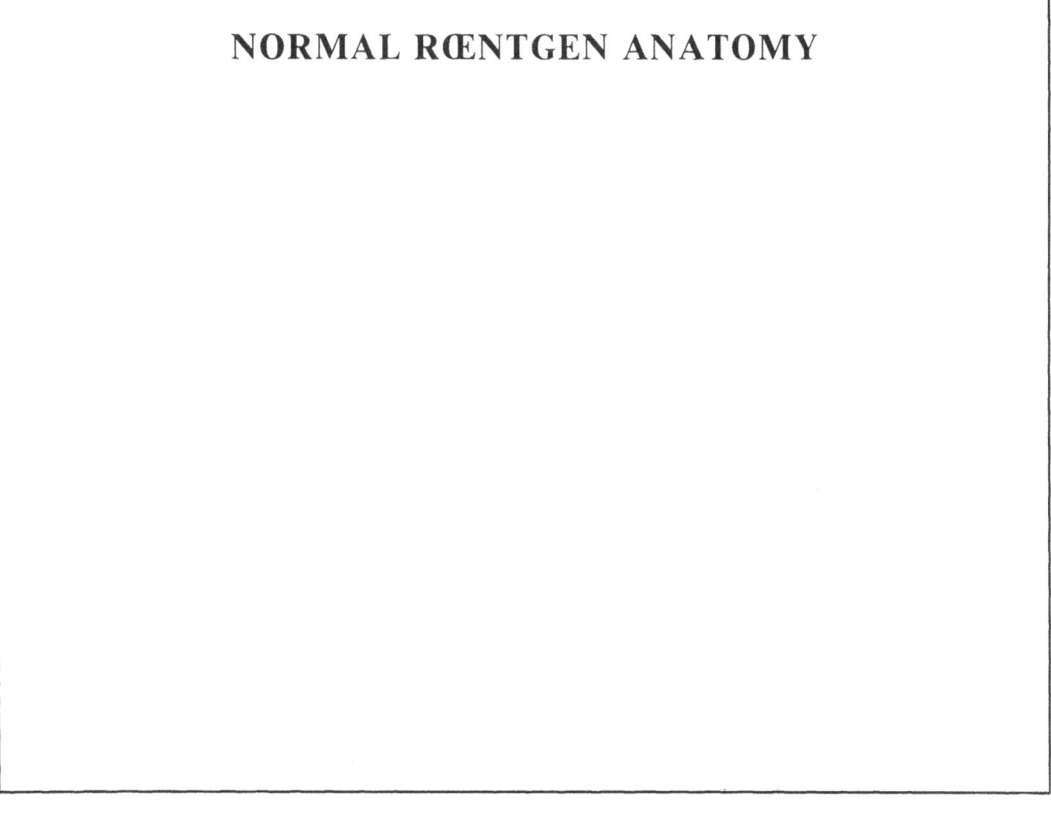

NORMAL RŒNTGEN ANATOMY

The rœntgen anatomy of the internal iliac artery and its branches is quite complex because of the number of these branches, their variations, the areas of distribution, and the great variety of planes in which they are localized. For the study of each of these arteries there exists one or two elective views which allow to expose it and to free it from disturbing superpositions.

We will discuss the rœntgen anatomy of the internal iliac artery and of its branches in the plane of election of the internal pudendal artery. In this oblique view not all arteries are visible. Only the internal iliac, iliolumbar, obturator, superior and inferior gluteal, and internal pudendal arteries and certain of the latter's branches can be identified.

I) INTERNAL ILIAC ARTERY

Origin

The internal iliac artery (hypogastric artery) arises from the common iliac artery of which it is the medial branch of bifurcation at the level of the bodies of the fifth lumbar and first sacral vertebrae and the intervening lumbosacral disk. The upper and lower extremes of the levels observed are the intervertebral space L4-5 and the body of S2, respectively. In a given individual the left and right internal iliac arteries originate at the same level in the majority of cases.

Course

The length of the rœntgenographic projection of the internal iliac artery is variable. It usually varies between 3.5 and 6 cm, the extremes being 2 and 10 cm. The artery courses obliquely in a caudal and posterior direction and presents a slight cephalad concavity.

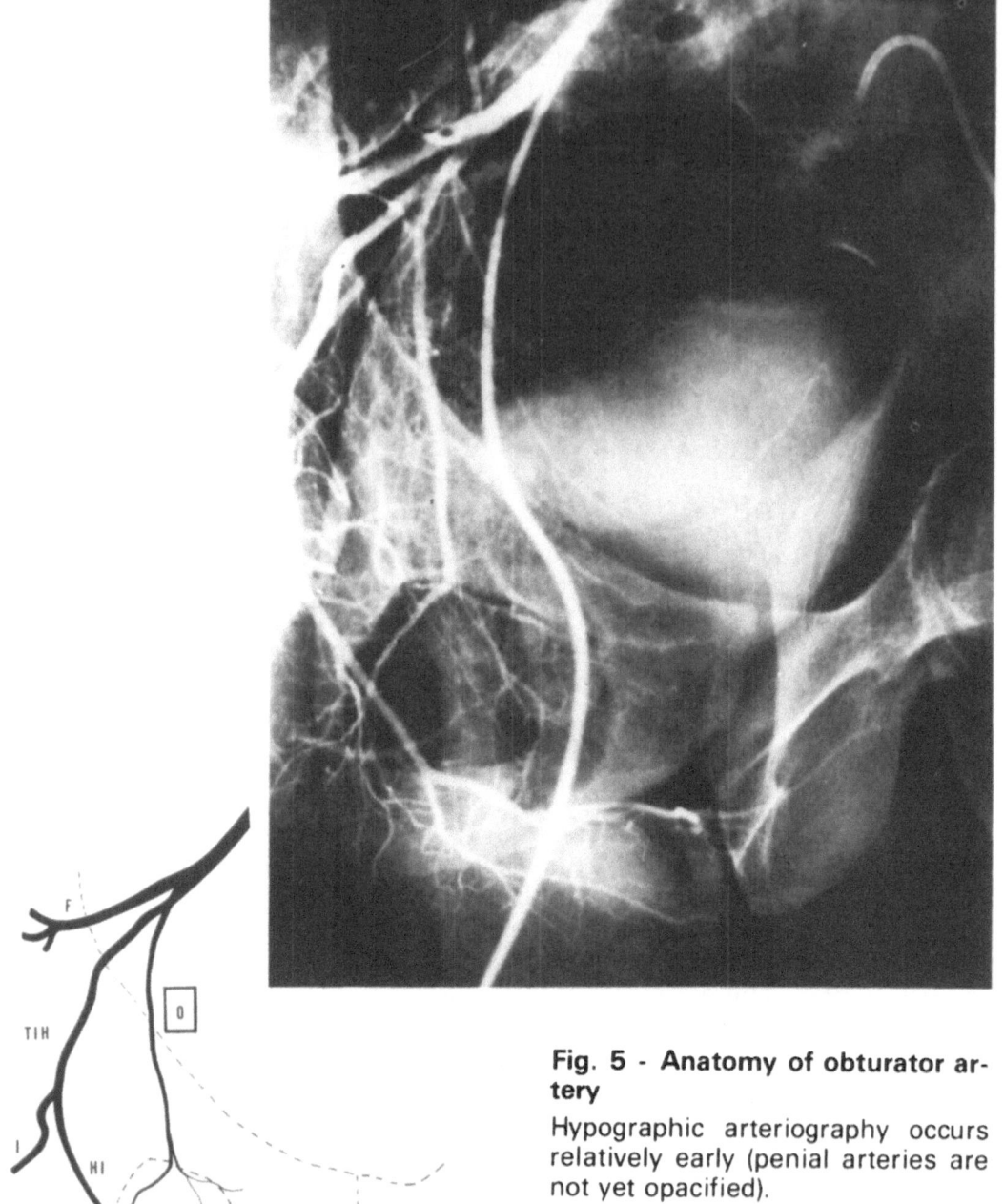

Fig. 5 - Anatomy of obturator artery

Hypographic arteriography occurs relatively early (penial arteries are not yet opacified).

Obturator artery arising from trifurcation of hypogastric artery in glutea artery, ischio-pudendal trunk and obturator artery.

Obturator arterial ring is easily seen.

Division

The end of the internal iliac artery is projected between the interspace S1-2 and the body of S3. The upper and lower extremes are the bodies of S1 and S4, respectively. Because of the oblique incidence it is not possible to correctly measure the distance between the end of the artery and the median plane.

There is a great variety in the types of division. In most cases the artery is divided into two trunks as follows.

— *The upper trunk,* called the posterior division, courses obliquely and laterally and usually gives off four branches : iliolumbar, superior lateral sacral, inferior lateral sacral, and superior gluteal arteries.

— *The lower trunk,* called the anterior division, courses obliquely down and laterally and divides into the following branches : obturator, umbilical, inferior gluteal, internal pudendal, inferior vesical, middle rectal, prostatic, and deferential (vesiculodeferential) arteries.

II) SUPERIOR GLUTEAL ARTERY

This largest of the branches of the internal iliac artery supplies the gluteal muscles. It can be divided into three segments.

● *The proximal segment* is oblique downward and laterally. It is projected above the common stem of the inferior gluteal and internal pudendal arteries, forming with it an acute angle. Its length depends upon the level at which the internal iliac artery ends.

● *The middle segment* is short, has an upward directed concavity, and corresponds to the passage of the superior gluteal artery below the upper border of the greater sciatic notch.

● *The distal, or gluteal, segment.*

The terminal branches of the superior gluteal artery, a superficial branch for the gluteus maximus muscle, and a deep branch for the medius and minimus muscles, cannot always be distinguished from each other. In this view, the aspect is in most cases that of an arborization or terminal bouquet.

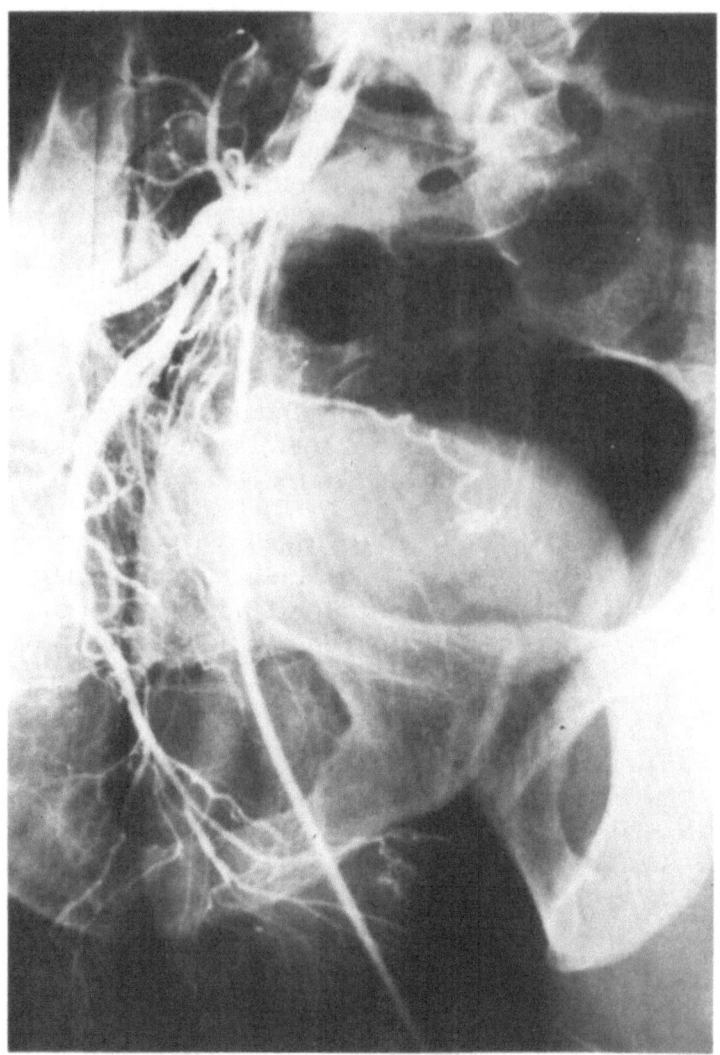

Fig. 6-7 - Variations of origins of obturator artery

Obturator artery is not seen on hypogastric arteriography.

Atheromatous stenoses are present on perineal part of internal pudendal artery and on superficial perineal. Penial dorsal deep arteries are amputated from their origin.

Selective epigastric arteriography shows that obturator artery arises from a common trunk with this latter.

Anastomosis between anterior and posterior branches of obturator is easily seen.

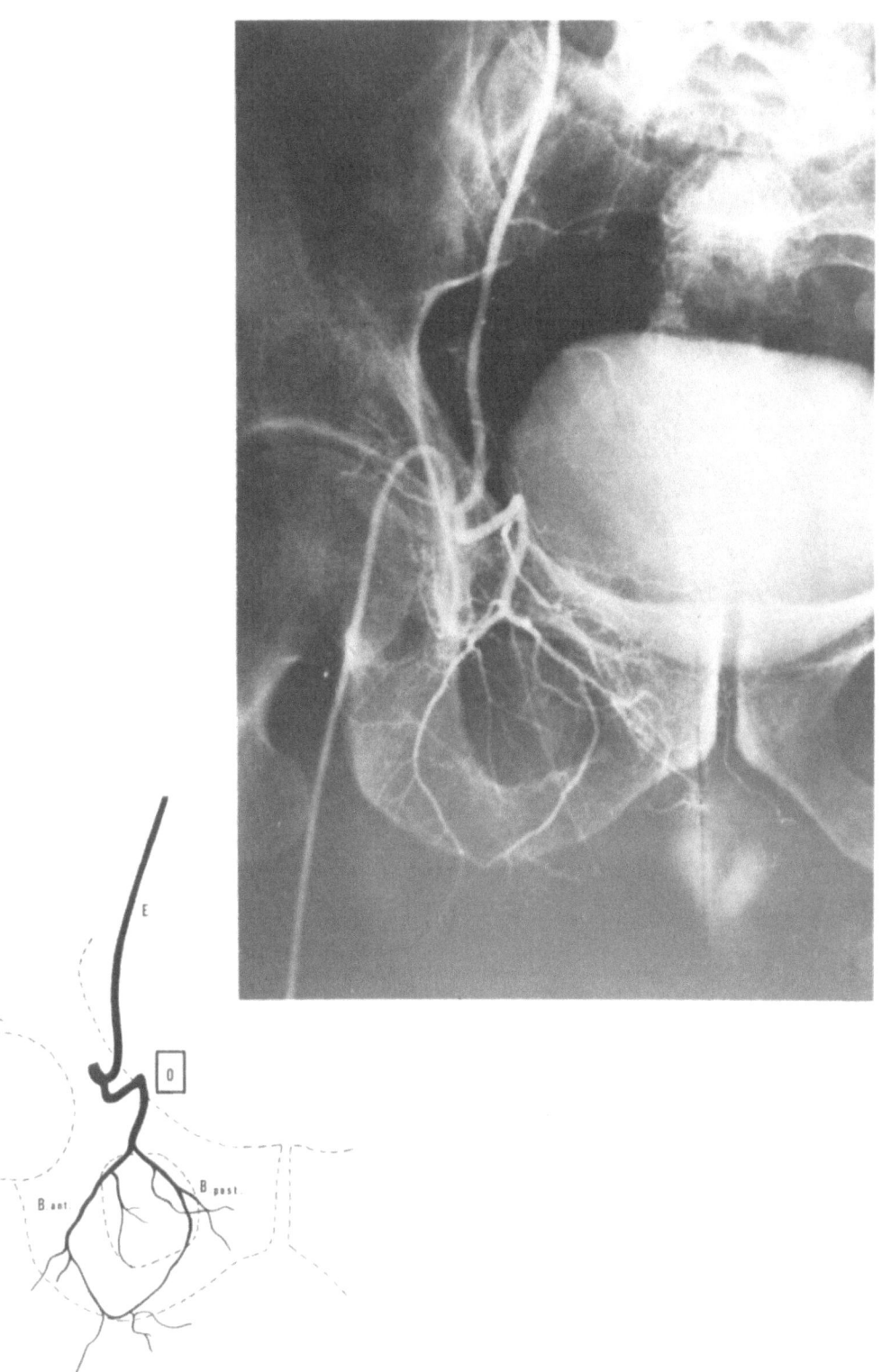

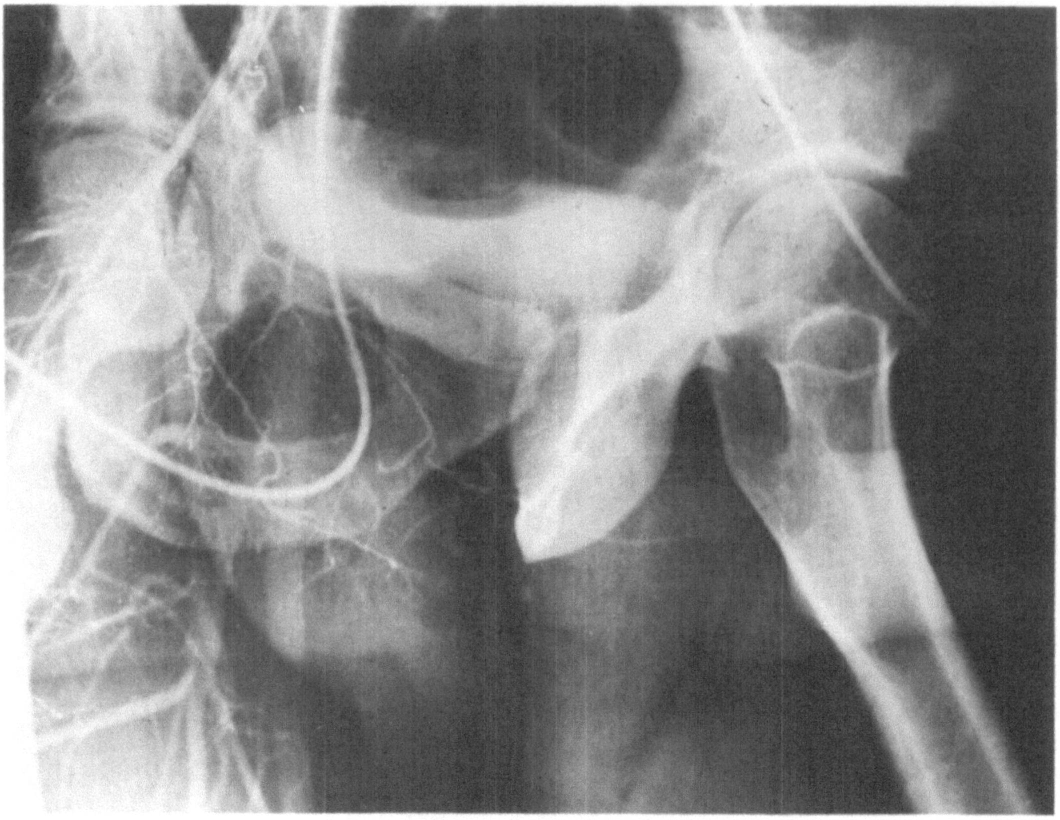

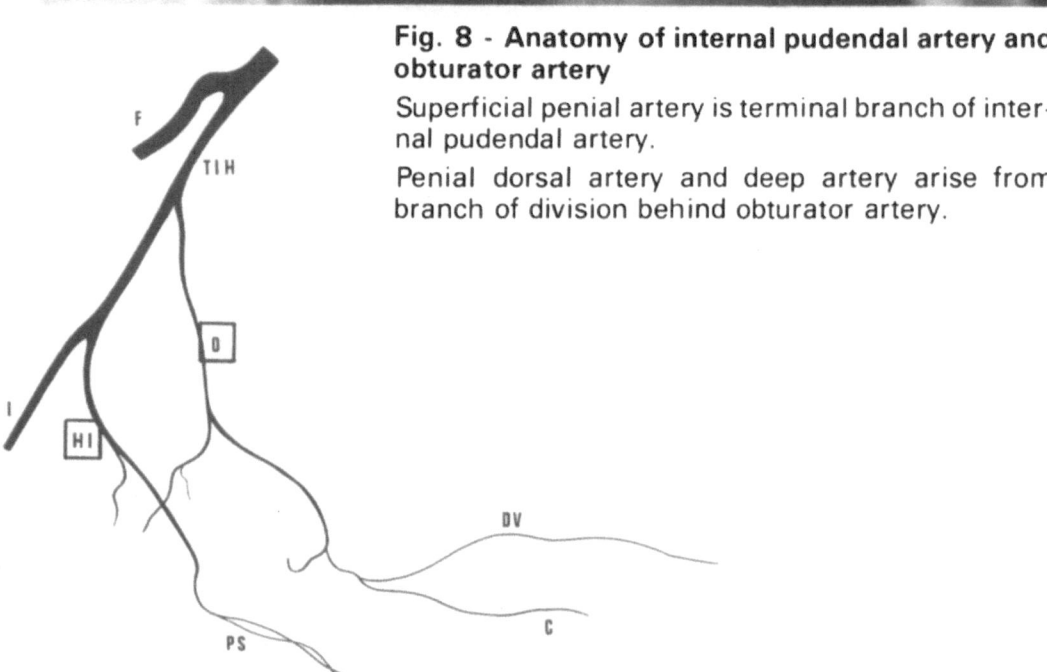

Fig. 8 - Anatomy of internal pudendal artery and obturator artery

Superficial penial artery is terminal branch of internal pudendal artery.

Penial dorsal artery and deep artery arise from branch of division behind obturator artery.

III) ILIOLUMBAR ARTERY

Almost always visible, the iliolumbar artery arises from the upper border of the internal iliac artery or the superior gluteal artery. Usually, if the internal iliac is relatively long, it is from that artery that the iliolumbar originates ; otherwise it springs from the superior gluteal artery.

IV) COMMUN TRUNK OF INFERIOR GLUTEAL AND INTERNAL PUDENDAL ARTERIES

This vascular segment is straight, continuing in most cases the direction of the internal iliac artery. Its length depends upon the level at which the internal iliac artery ends and the level at which the trunk divides into the two vessels. Its division can be as low as the level of the ischial spine, i.e. in the area of its passage of the greater sciatic notch. Between this lowermost limit of the division of the common trunk and its complete absence (terminal bouquet of the internal iliac artery) all intermediary levels have been observed.

V) INFERIOR GLUTEAL ARTERY

Only the proximal segment of the inferior gluteal artery is visualized in this view. It is straight, continuing the direction of the stem that it shares with the internal pudendal artery. Its projection is seen above the proximal segment of the internal pudendal artery.

Sometimes the inferior gluteal artery originates from a trunk it has in common with the superior gluteal artery, or it may arise directly from the internal iliac artery, participating in the latter's terminal bouquet.

VI) OBTURATOR ARTERY

Origin

Most often the obturator artery is a branch — direct or indirect — of the internal iliac artery. It may however also arise from the inferior epigastric *, the external iliac, or the femoral artery. In

---

* In this case, the artery takes the name of accessory obturator artery (Translator's note).

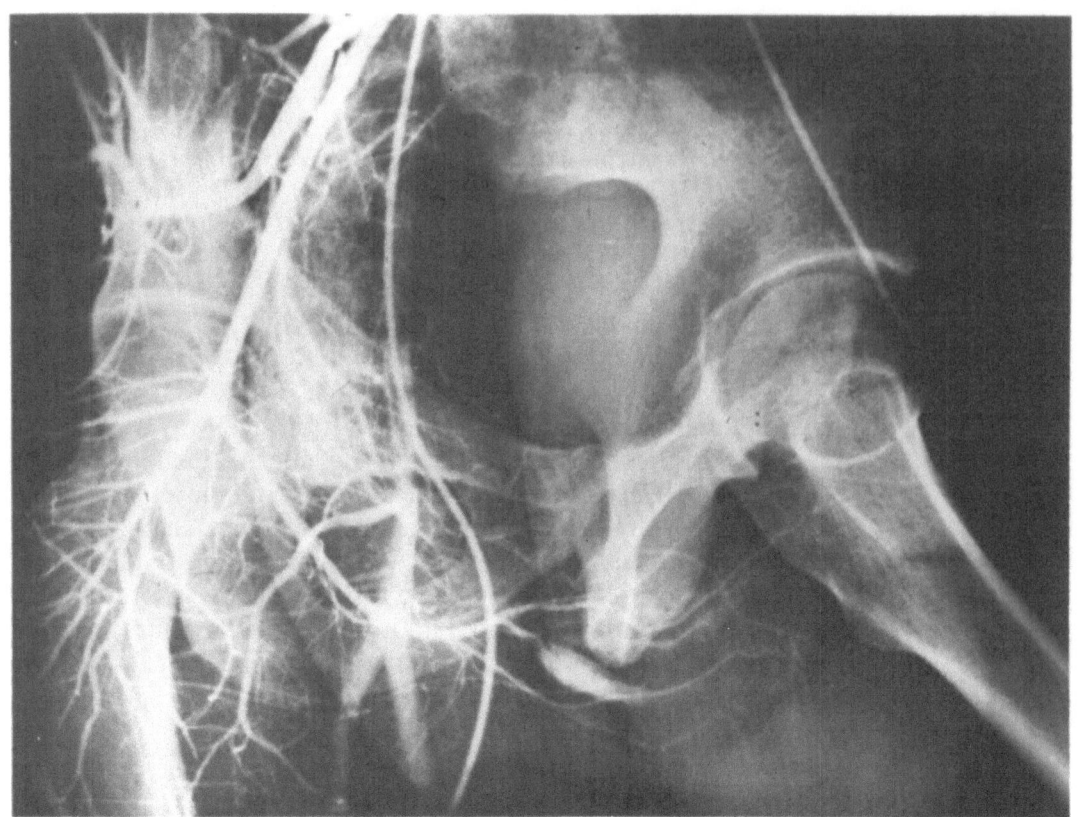

Fig. 9-10 - Normal anatomy of internal pudendal artery

Internal pudendal artery arises at level of ischial spine.

Its ischio-rectal part and perineal part are easily seen.

Superficial perineal artery arises at level of ischio-pubien branch. Only internal branch is individualizable.

Artery of penial bulb is voluminous and a parenchymatous time exists from the start of arterial time.

Deep artery is easily seen.

Dorsal artery projects above deep artery.

After a delay, presence of parenchymatous cavernosum and spongiosum.

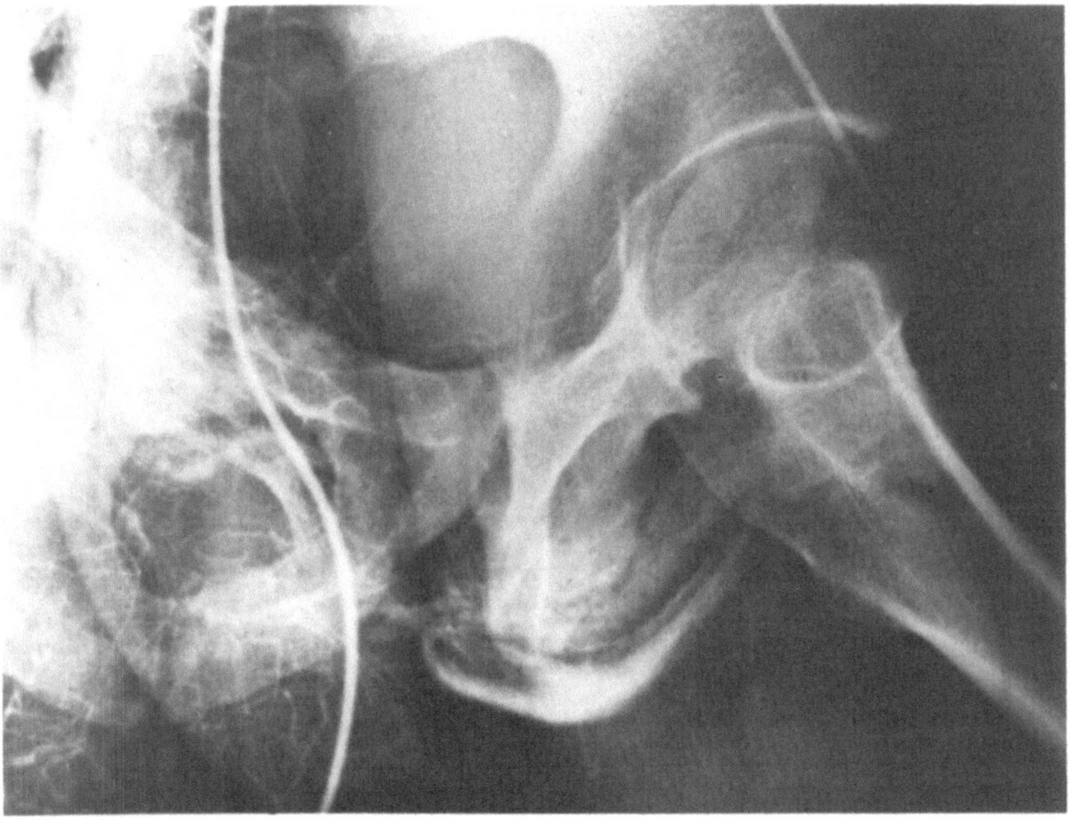

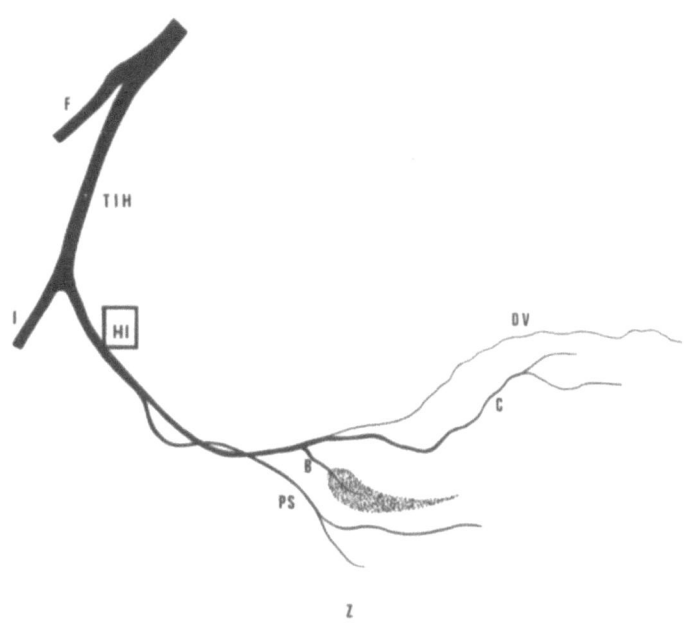

arteriography of internal pudendal artery/**37**

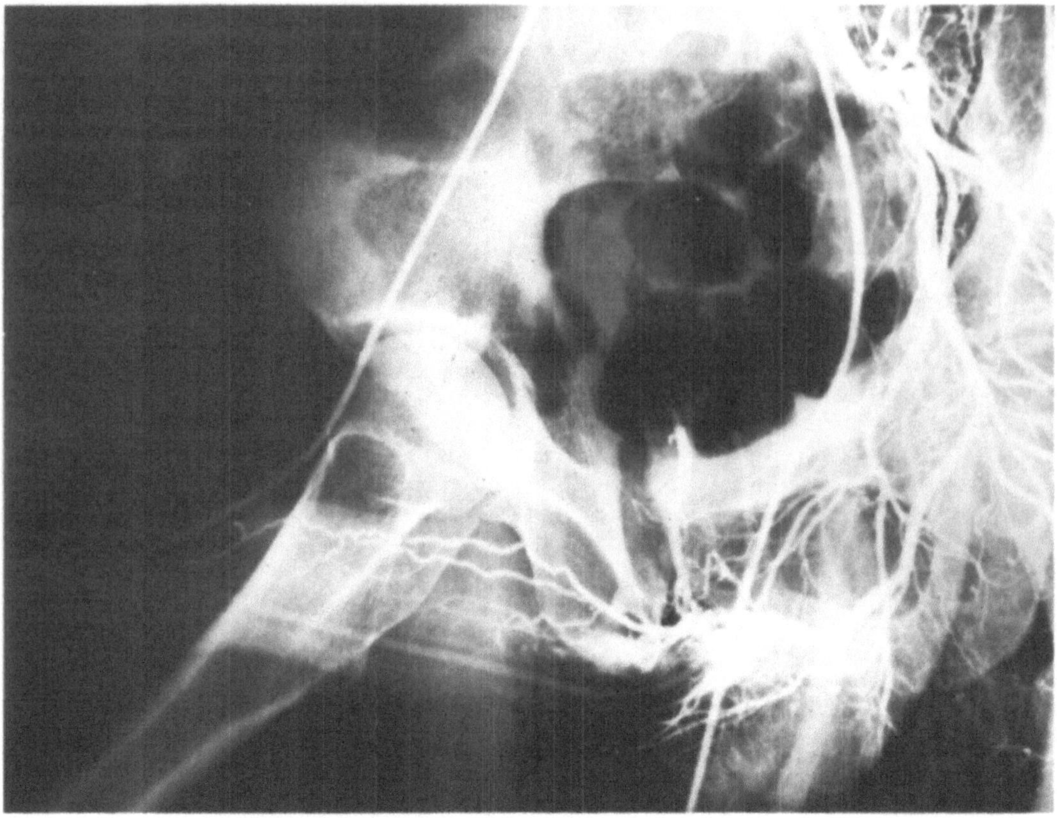

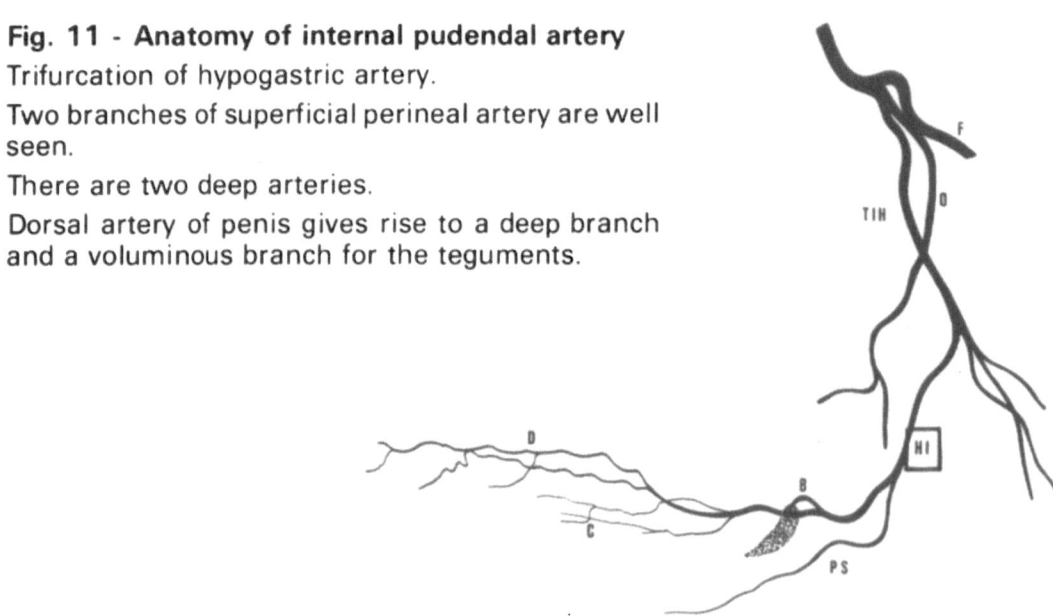

Fig. 11 - Anatomy of internal pudendal artery

Trifurcation of hypogastric artery.

Two branches of superficial perineal artery are well seen.

There are two deep arteries.

Dorsal artery of penis gives rise to a deep branch and a voluminous branch for the teguments.

our experience the obturator artery arises in 36 per cent of the cases from the common trunk of the inferior gluteal and the internal pudendal arteries ; in 30 per cent from the internal iliac artery, either as a side branch or as one of the branches of the terminal bouquet ; and in 12 per cent from the superior gluteal artery.

In selective arteriography of the internal iliac artery, the obturator artery is not visualized in 22 per cent of the cases. This group includes atypical origins of the obturator artery and cases where its anastomoses with the inferior epigastric artery are hemodynamically predominant.

Course

The obturator artery first forms a lateral concavity, then runs for several centimeters along the pelvic brim (linea terminalis) or a few centimeters above or below it. It then crosses the iliopubic ramus and reaches the upper border of the obturator foramen where it ends.

Among its branches, only the one to the internal obturator muscle is usually discernible. An anastomosis with the inferior epigastric artery is visualized in exceptional cases. The ascending, public or vesical branches are not visible or identifiable.

Division

The obturator artery terminates always at the same level, the upper border of the obturator foramen. It divides usually into two branches.

— The anterior, or internal, branch courses around the anterior half of the obturator foramen and gives off several muscular rami which are clearly visible.

— The posterior, or external, branch embraces the posterior half of the obturator foramen.

A third, the acetabular, branch is only rarely visualized. It opacifies with delay and at that stage numerous arteriolar opacifications interfer with its identification. For the same reason the anastomosis between the anterior and posterior branches, which completes the arterial circle around the obturator foramen, is not often visible.

In 10 per cent of the cases the branch destined for the adductor muscles is quite large. In two per cent of the cases the artery terminates in a trifurcation, the third branch being the artery of the adductor muscles. In two cases the obturator artery gave origin to the dorsal and deep arteries of the penis.

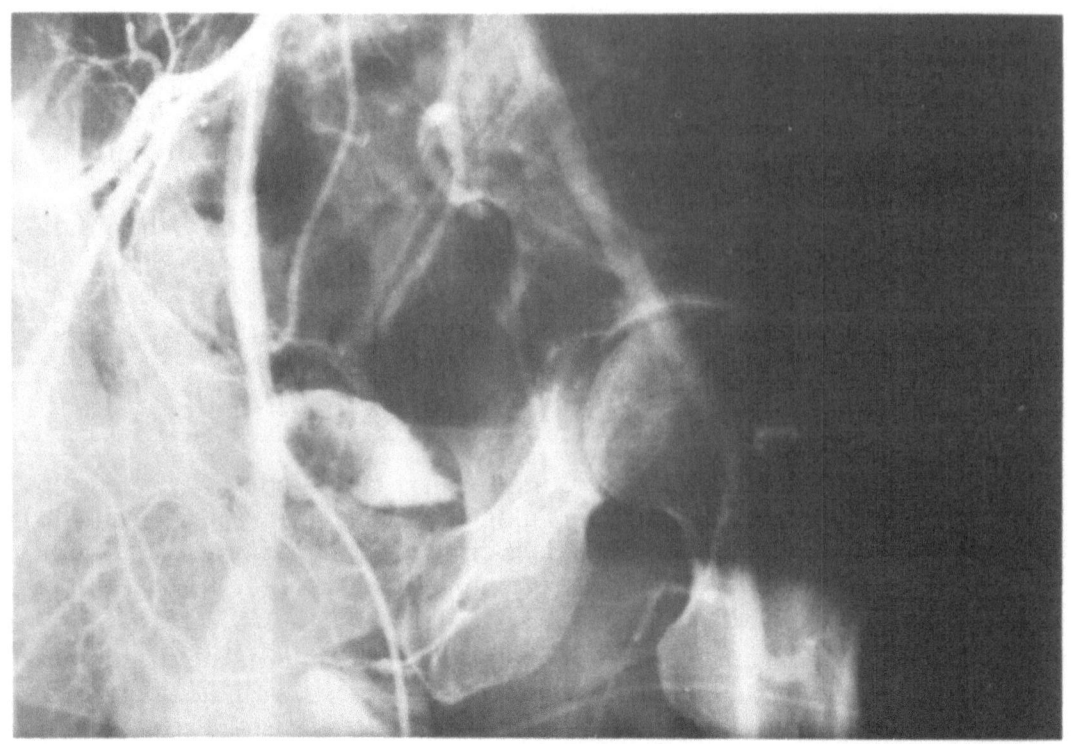

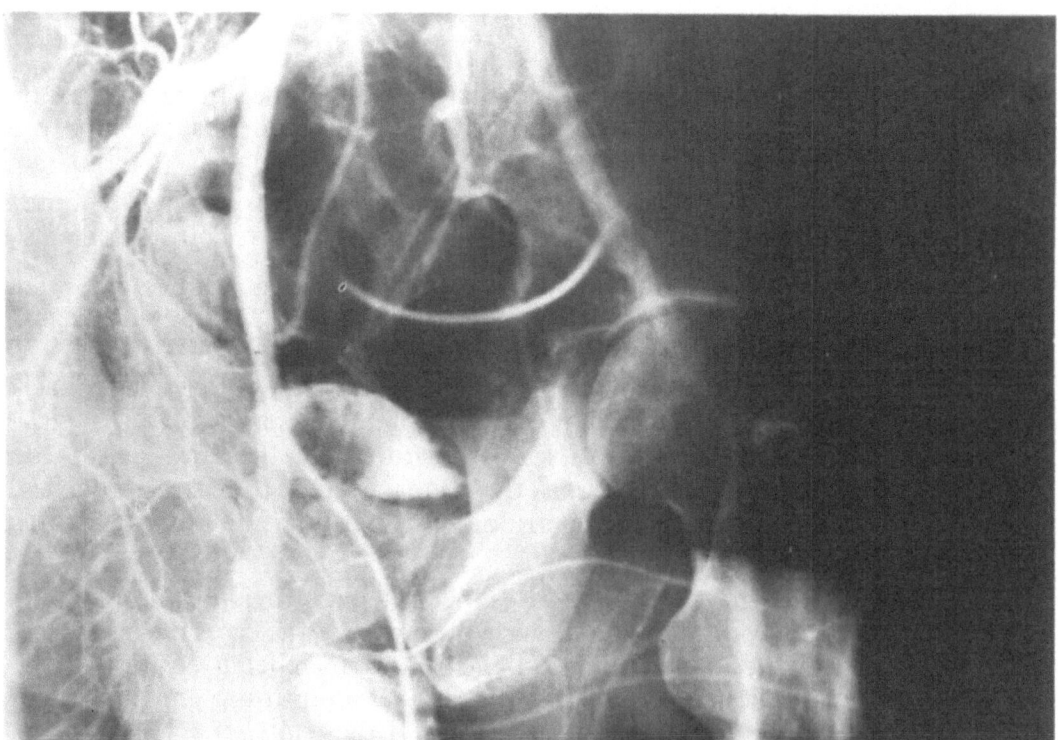

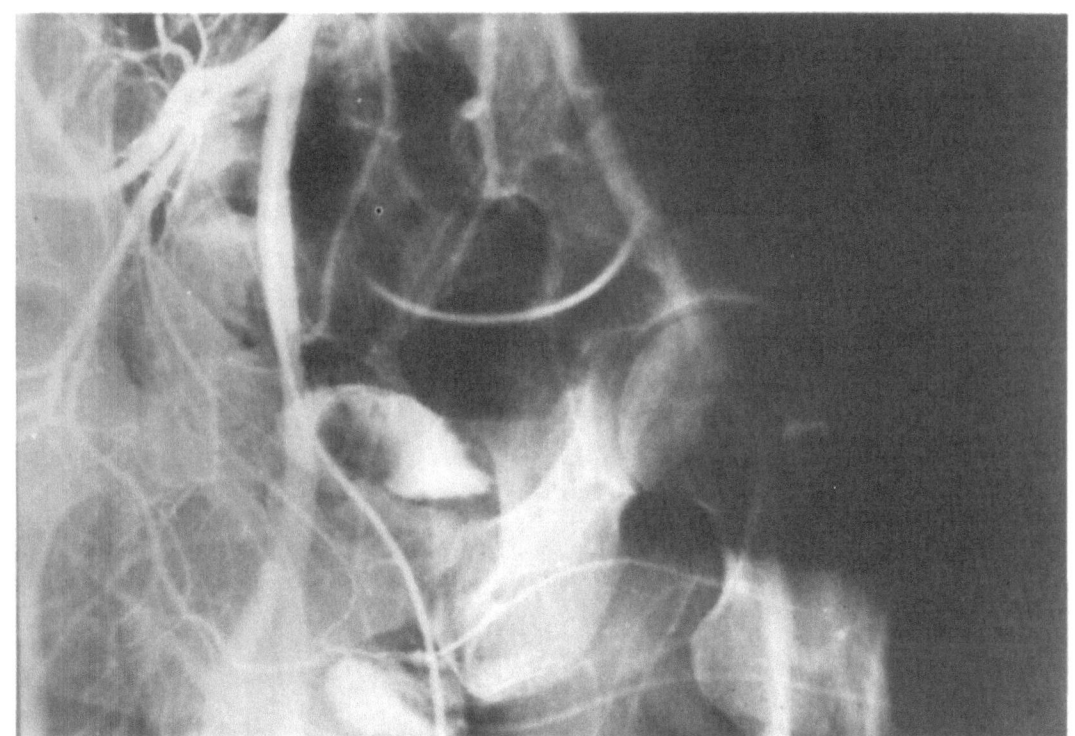

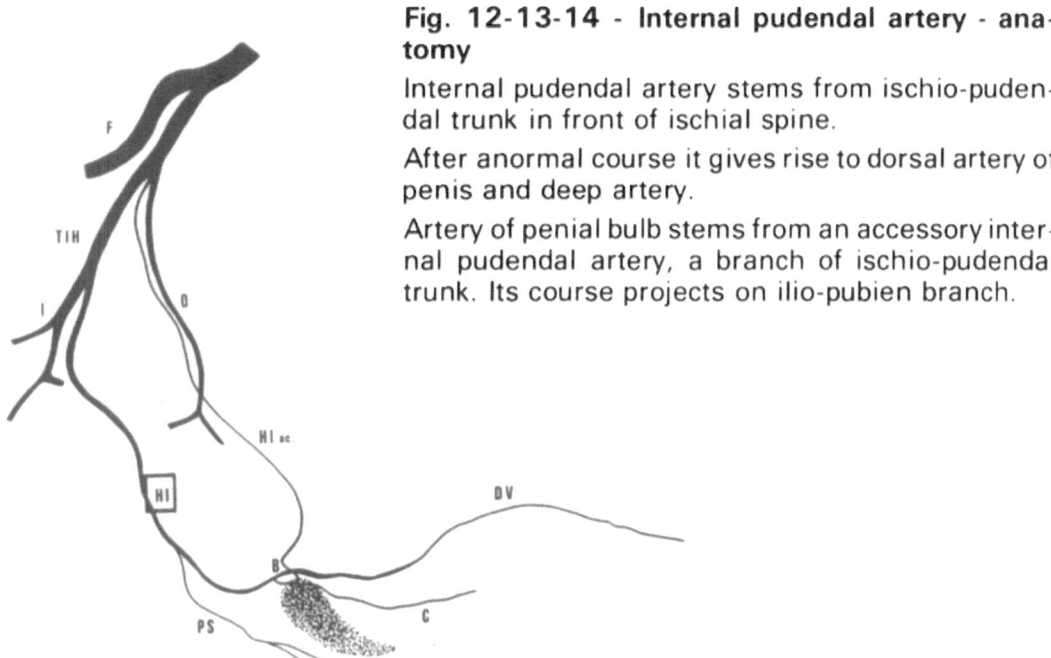

Fig. 12-13-14 - Internal pudendal artery - anatomy

Internal pudendal artery stems from ischio-pudendal trunk in front of ischial spine.

After anormal course it gives rise to dorsal artery of penis and deep artery.

Artery of penial bulb stems from an accessory internal pudendal artery, a branch of ischio-pudendal trunk. Its course projects on ilio-pubien branch.

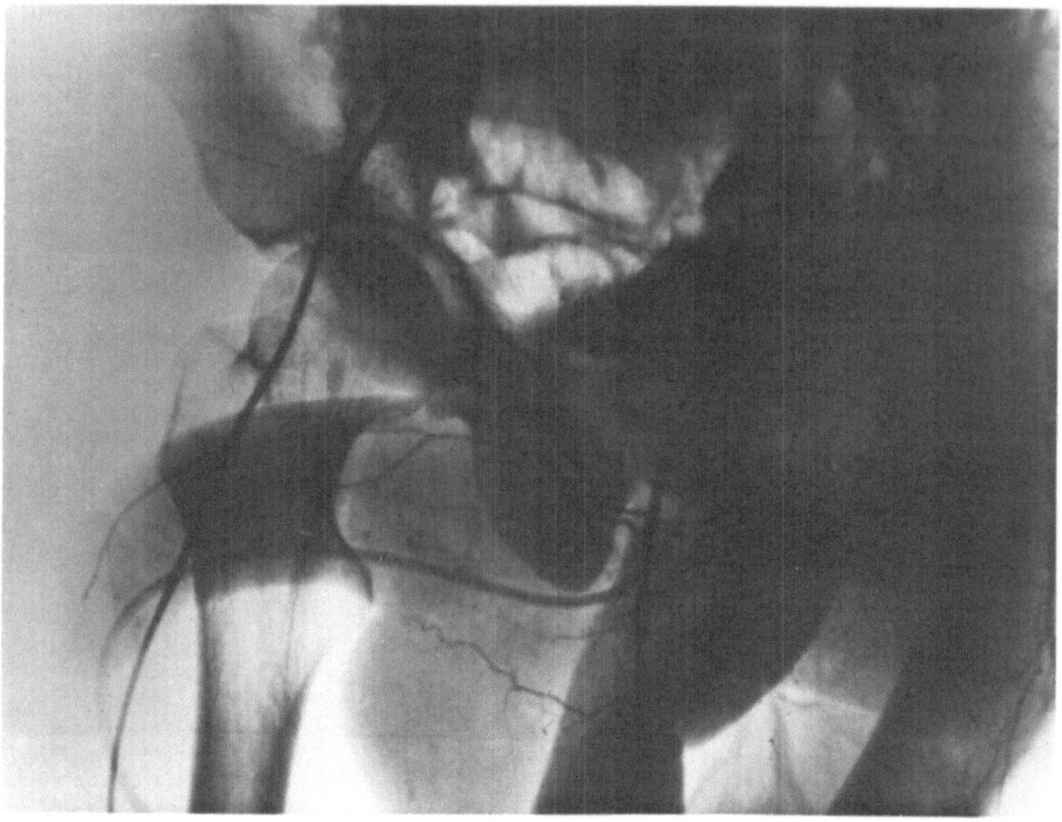

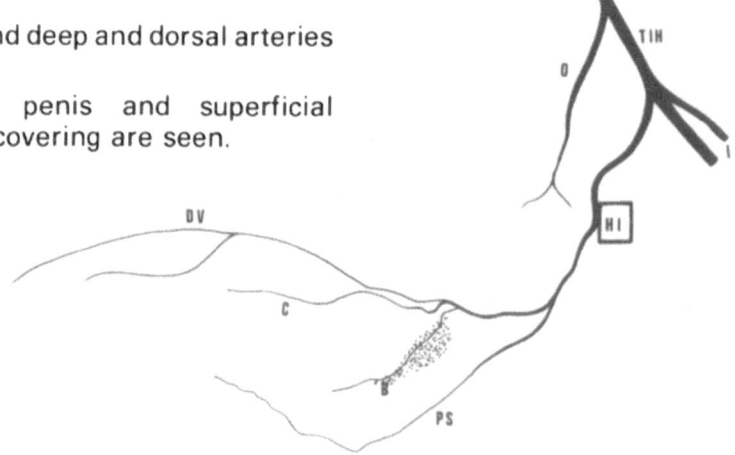

Fig. 15 - Normal anatomy of internal pudendal artery

Low division of ischio-pudendal trunk at level of ischial spine.

Penial arteries of bulb, and deep and dorsal arteries of penis are easily seen.

Circonflex arteries of penis and superficial branches for penis skin covering are seen.

This is the artery of the erectile organs. Some anatomists consider it to be the terminal branch of the internal iliac artery.

Origin

There is less variety in the origin of the internal pudendal than in that of the obturator artery. In our series the internal pudendal artery arises in 73 per cent of the cases from the trunk it shares with the inferior gluteal artery, a trunk which sometimes is extremely short; in 14 per cent of the cases from a terminal bouquet (arborization) of the internal iliac artery; and in 11 per cent of the cases from a terminal trifurcation of the internal iliac artery. This trifurcation can be one of two patterns, grouping either superior gluteal, inferior gluteal, and internal pudental arteries, or common trunk of gluteal arteries, internal pudendal, and obturator arteries. (The most frequent pattern of trifurcation of the internal iliac artery does not include the internal pudendal artery itself; it consists only of the trunk the latter has in common with the inferior gluteal artery, the superior gluteal, and the obturator arteries).

The level of origin of the internal pudendal artery shows great variations. It extends from the end of the internal iliac artery (terminal bouquet or trifurcation) as far as the low division of the common gluteopudendal trunk, i.e. the level of the ischial spine (30 per cent of the cases).

Course

In the radiologic anatomy of the internal pudendal artery four segments can be recognized : pelvic, gluteal, ischiorectal and perineal.

● *The pelvic segment :*

It is oblique downward and posteriorly, slightly concave downward and anteriorly. The artery takes the direction of the ischial spine. In those cases where the internal pudendal separates itself at a low level from the trunk it shares with the inferior gluteal, this segment is either very short or nonexistant.

● *The gluteal segment :*

It is very short. This is the segment that forms a loop around the ischial spine. Radiologically it presents itself as a change in the direction of the internal pudendal artery. The arc it makes is more or less open.

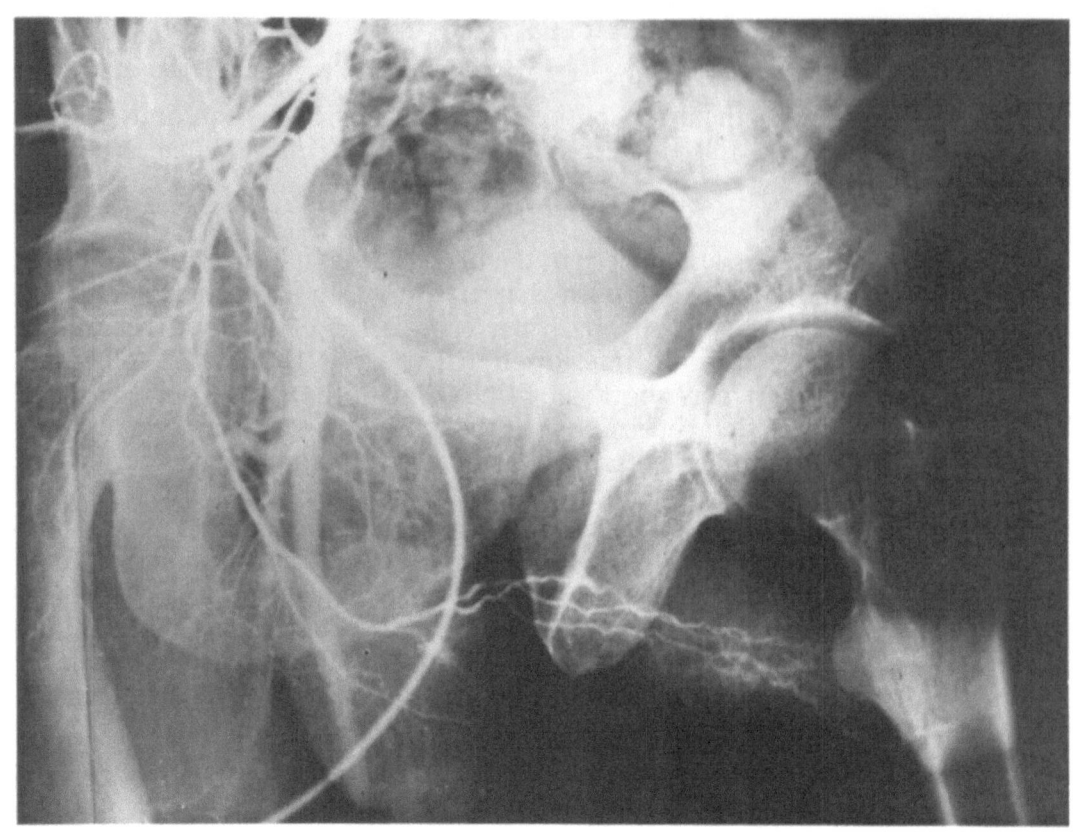

Fig. 16-17 - Normal anatomy of penial arteries

When penis is not placed at precise profile position, dorsal artery of penis and deep artery are superimposed and not easily dissociable.

After delay of time, good cavernography.

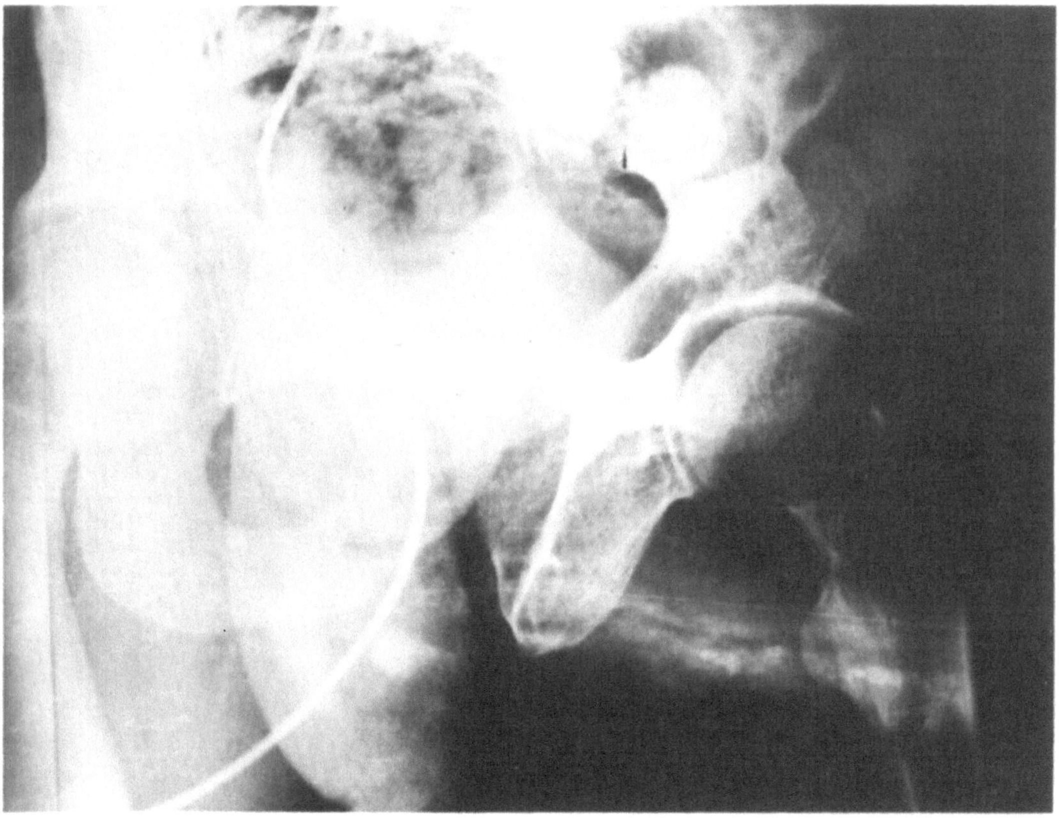

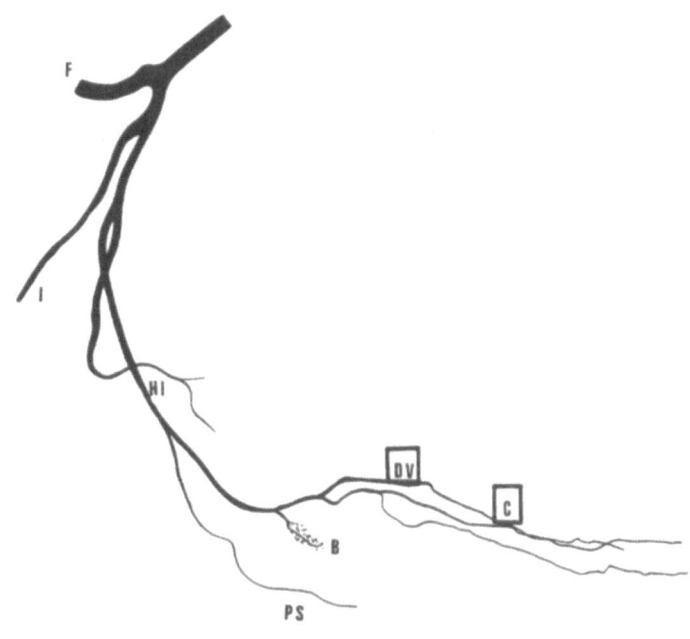

arteriography of internal pudendal artery/**45**

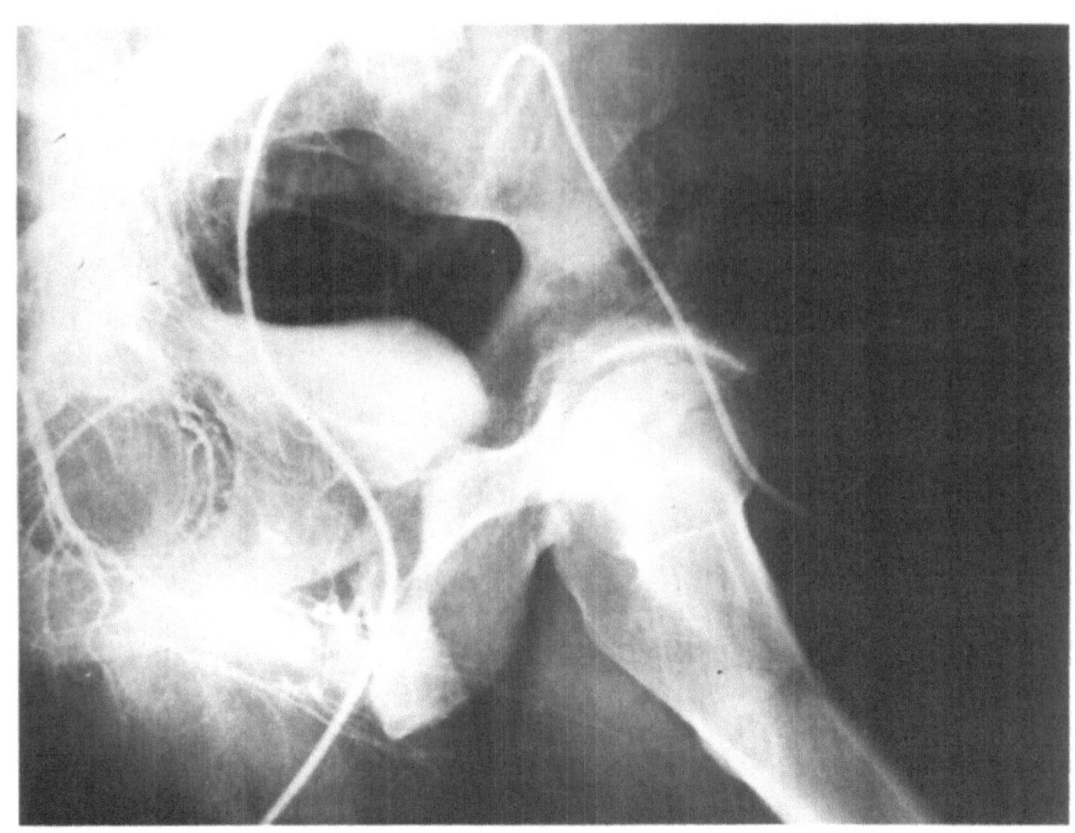

Fig. 18-19 - Anatomy of deep artery
Presence of several rectilinear deep arteries, smaller than normal.
After delay of time, normal cavernogram.

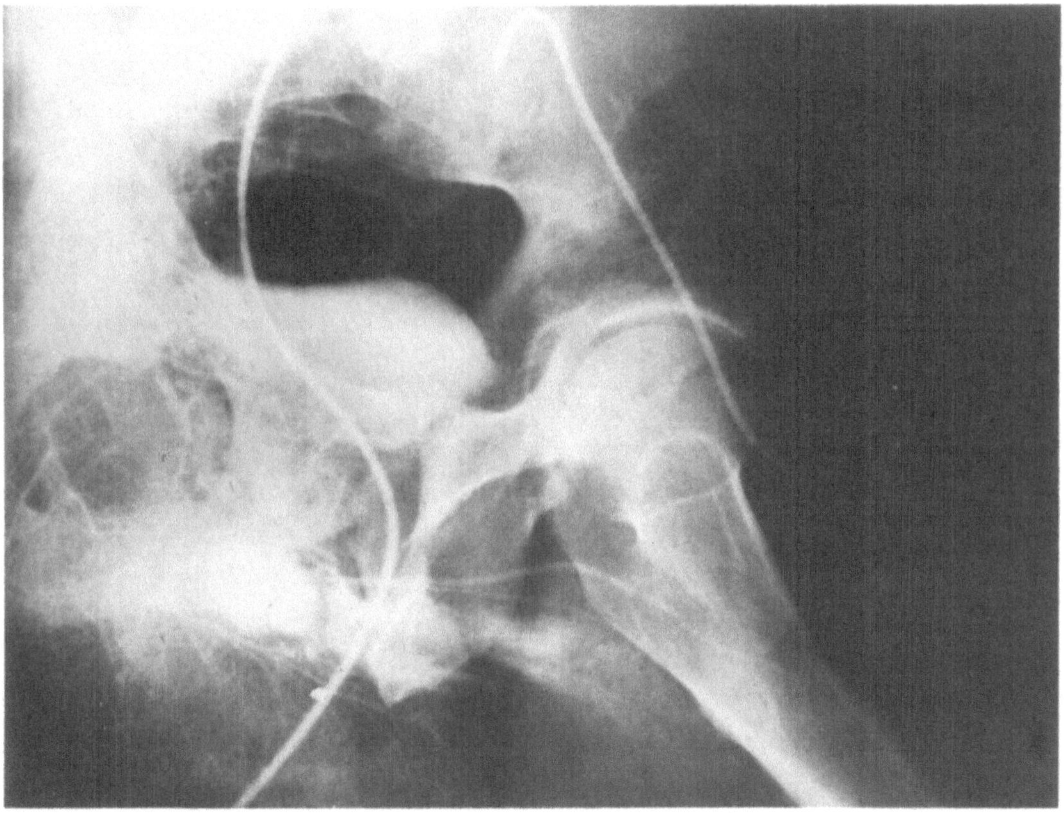

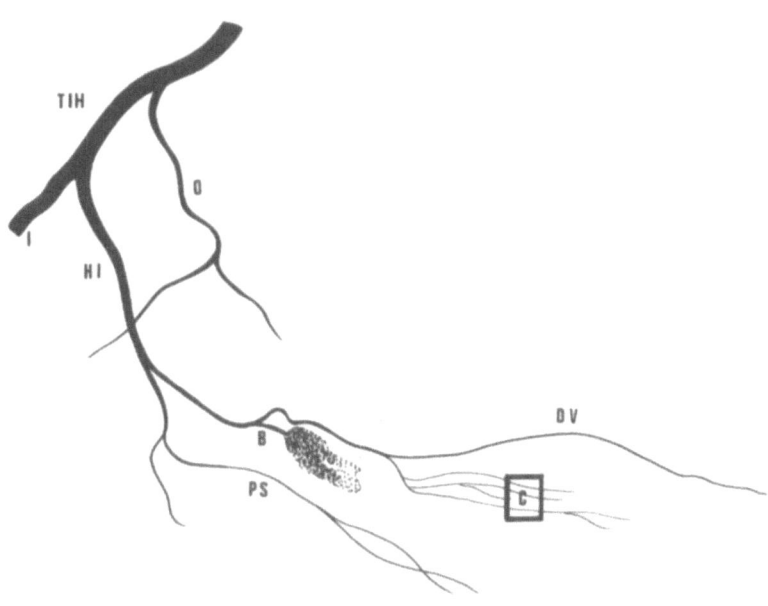

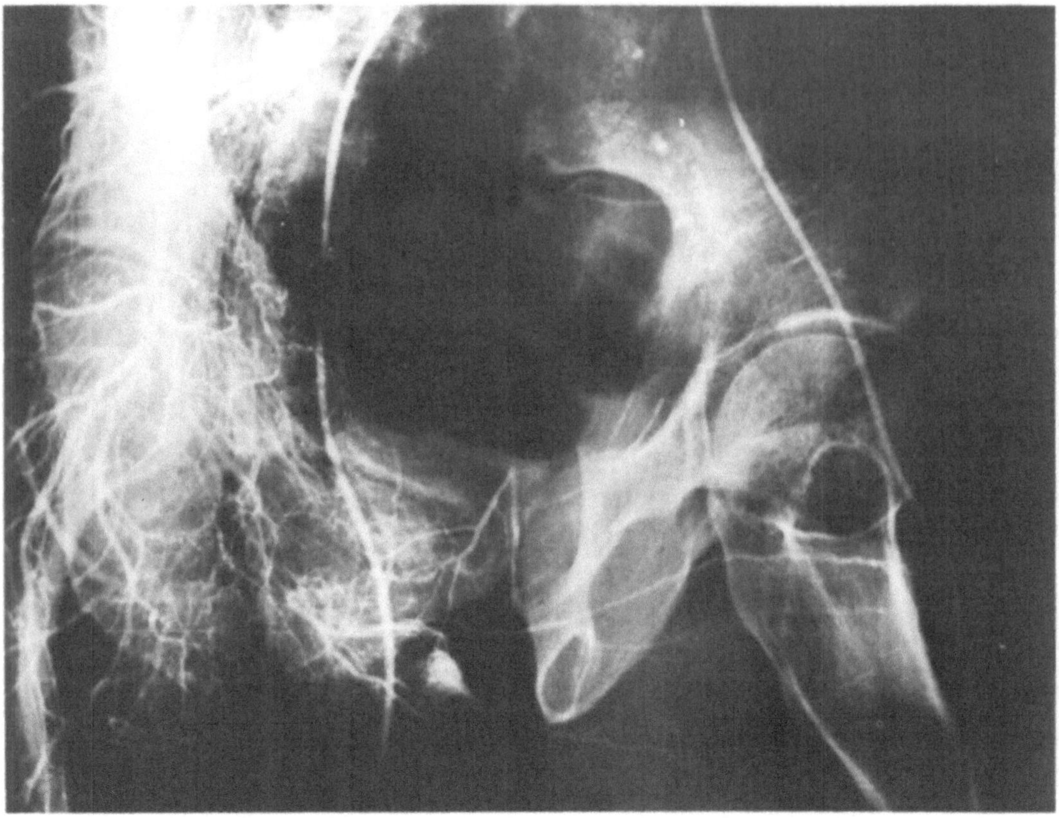

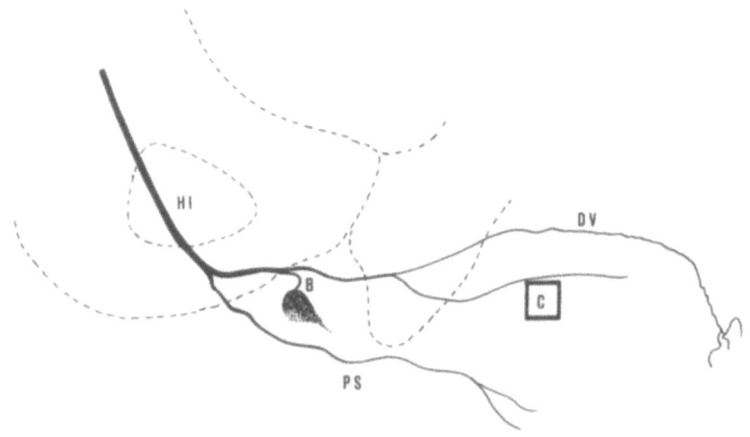

Fig. 20 - Anatomy of deep artery

Late origin of deep artery further along the sub-pubien arch.

Circonflex arteries are easily seen.

- *The ischiorectal segment :*

It is comprised between the point where the internal pudendal passes the lesser sciatic notch and the point where it enters the perineum. Its course is roughly straight, its direction exactly oblique downward and anteriorly, and its length is rather constant, i.e. between 6 and 8 cm.

- *The perineal segment :*

Courses anteriorly and slightly upward along the ischiopubic ramus as far as the pubic arch. This relationship with the ischiopubic ramus is very important. The internal pudendal artery is indeed the only artery which at some time is superimposed upon the ischiopubic ramus. When it is difficult to distinguish the upper segment from other pelvic arteries, it is by following this segment that the internal pudendal artery can be identified.

Branches

Muscular branches and visceral branches of small volumes destined for the rectum, the prostate and the bladder cannot be distinguished.

- *Inferior rectal arteries*

These cannot be recognized in this projection.

- *Perineal (superficial perineal) artery*

This is a large and constant branch. Its origin is projected to an area at the level of the lower part of the obturator foramen, the upper border of the ischiopubic ramus, or the ischiopubic ramus itself. The conventional division into two branches, internal and external, is seen only in 80 per cent of the cases.

- *Artery of the bulb of the penis*

Its origin is projected on the pubis or under the pubic arch. It is short and relatively large and it runs downward. It is easily identified, because its opacification is accompanied by a stage of bulbar parenchyma, appearing as early as the arterial stage.

- *Urethral artery*

This branch arises anterior to the artery of the penile bulb. It is of very small caliber and is rarely visible on the arteriographs. It supplies the corpus cavernosum and is characterized by its projection below the urethra.

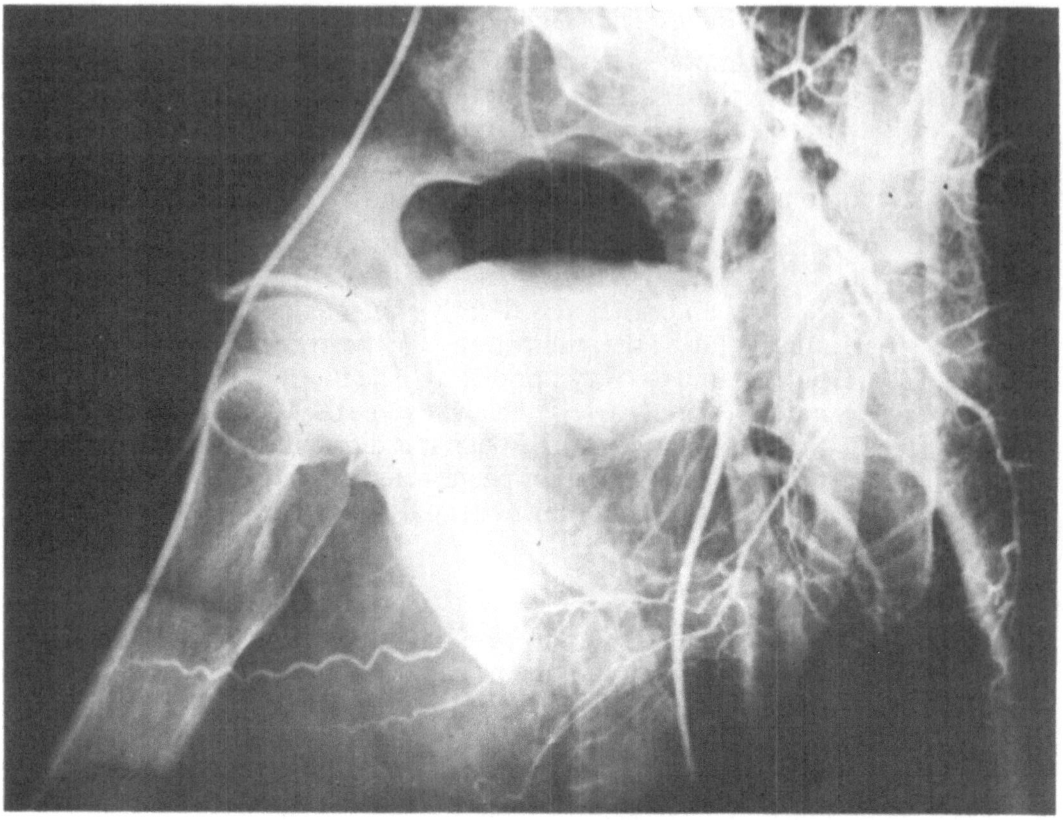

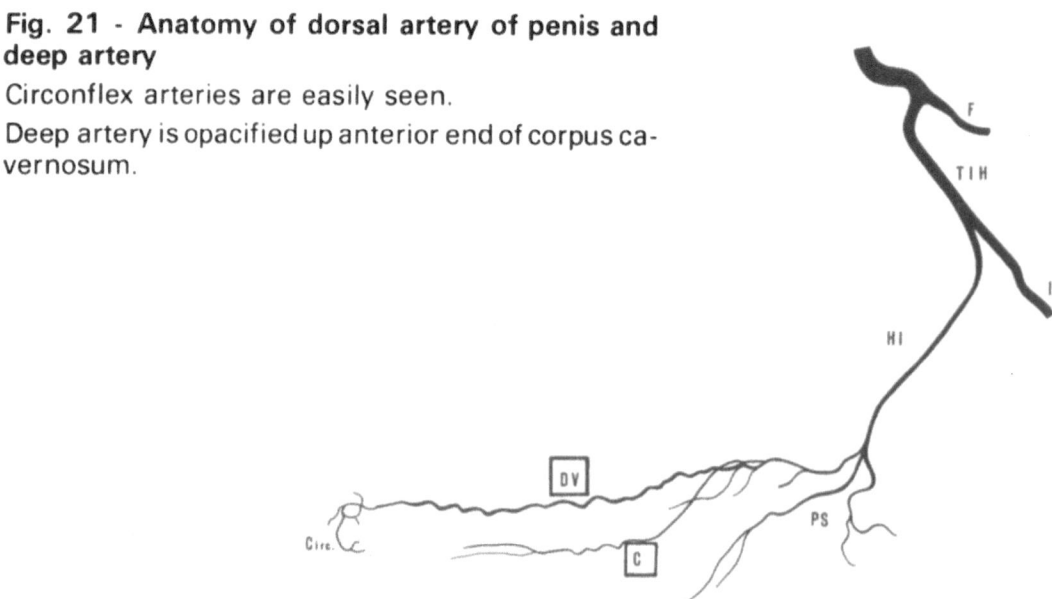

Fig. 21 - Anatomy of dorsal artery of penis and deep artery

Circonflex arteries are easily seen.

Deep artery is opacified up anterior end of corpus cavernosum.

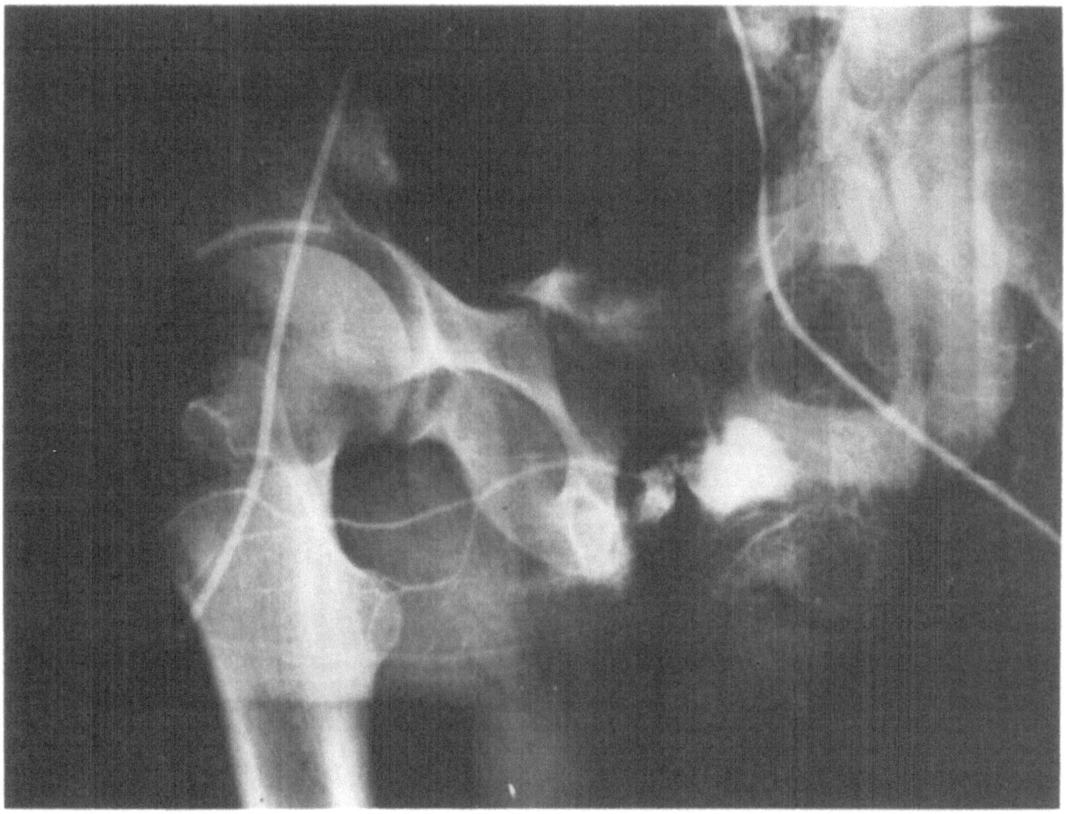

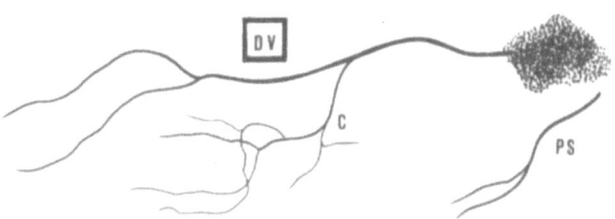

Fig. 22 - Anatomy of dorsal artery of penis

Dorsal artery gives rise to a voluminous deep branch.

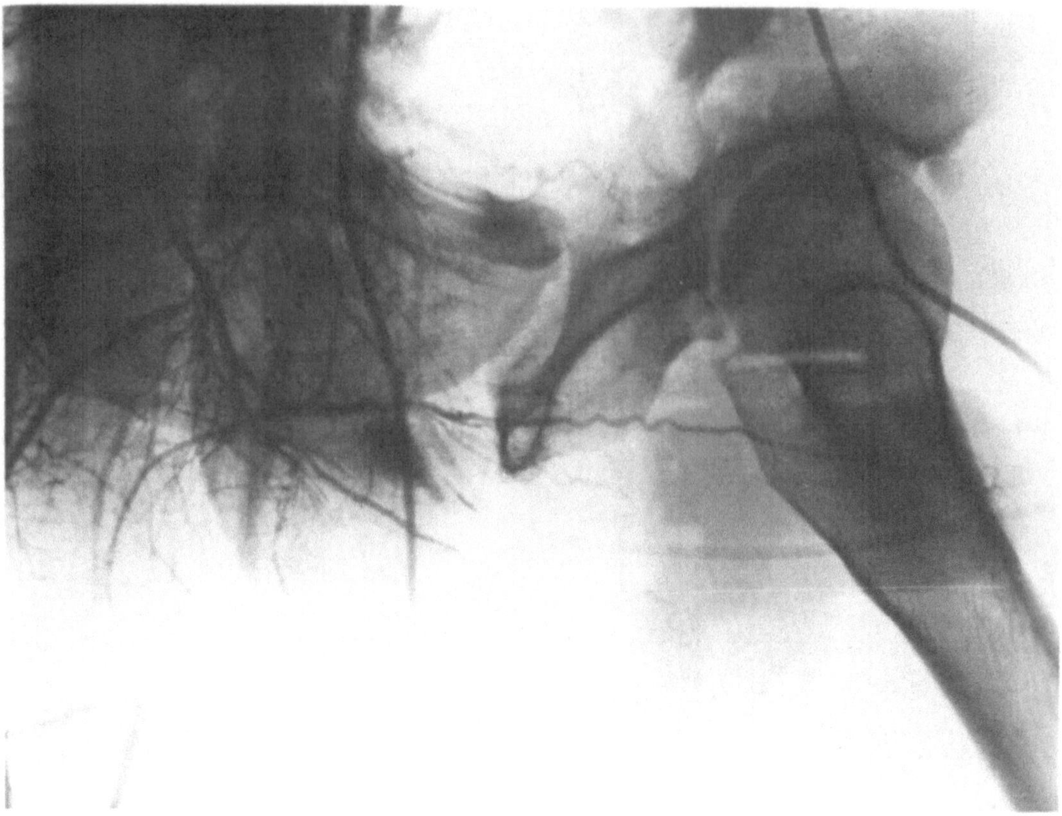

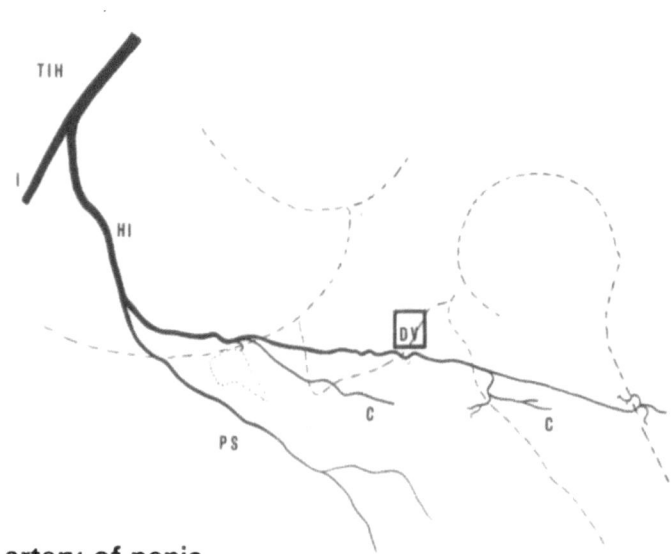

Fig. 23 - Anatomy of dorsal artery of penis
A deep branch (crossing in front of femur) is easily
seen.
Amputation of deep artery at medium third level.

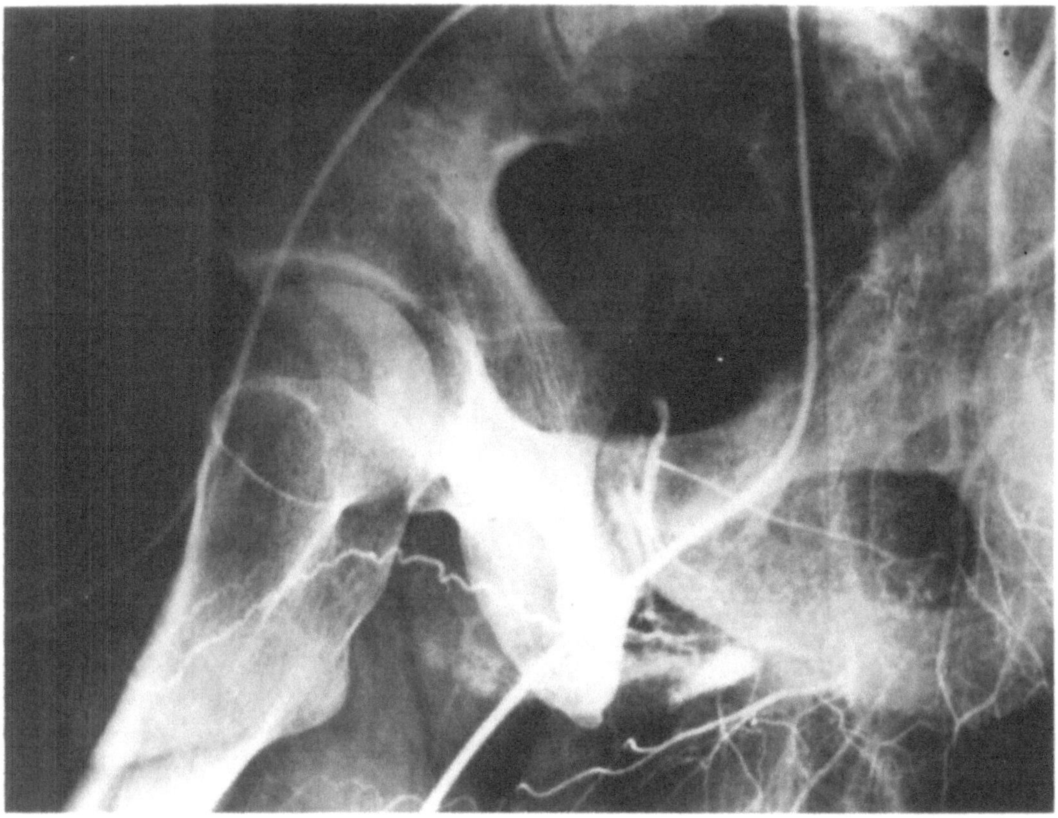

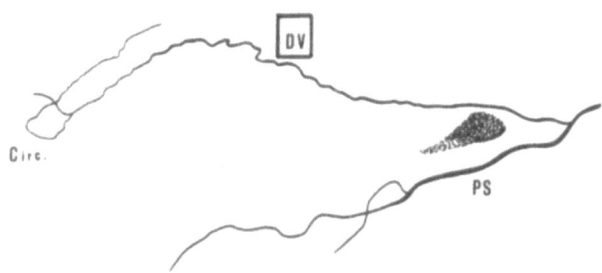

Fig. 24 - Anatomy of dorsal artery of penis

Retrograde opacification of end portion of dorsal artery of contralateral by circonflex ring.

This rarely occurs.

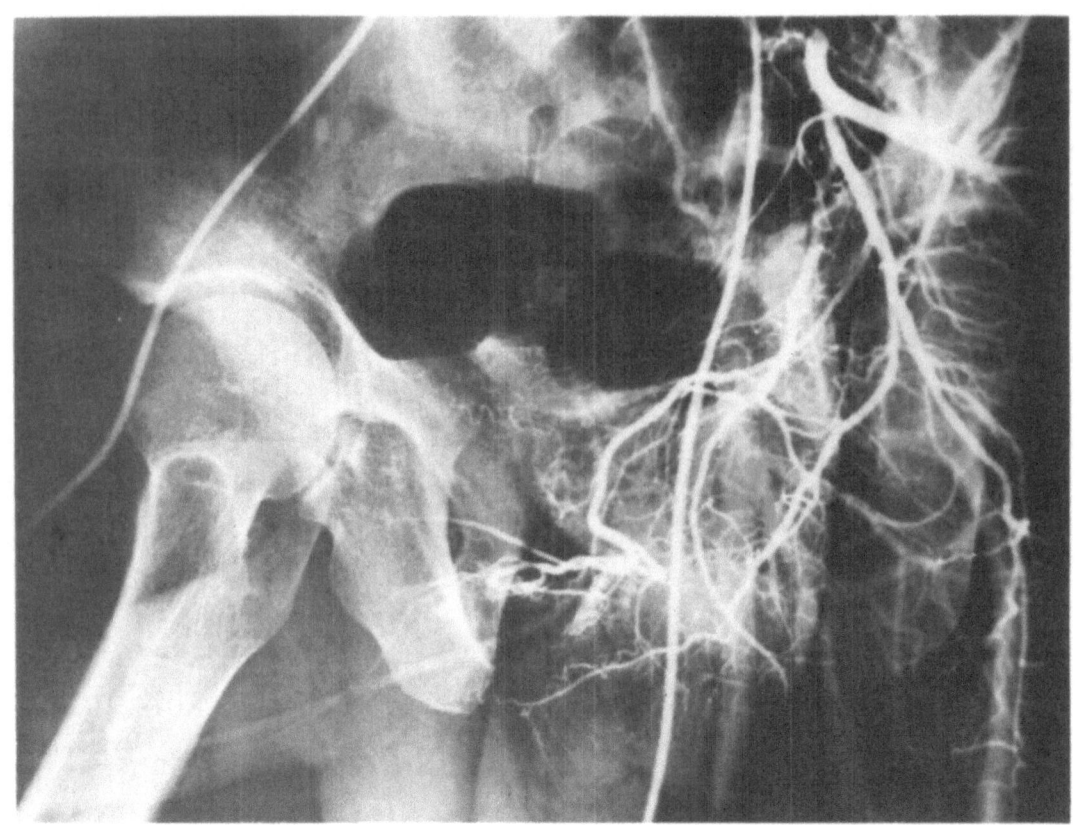

Fig. 25-26 - Accessory internal pudendal

The superficial perineal artery is the terminal artery of the internal pudendal.

An accessory internal pudendal artery, a branch of the ischio-pudendal trunk, runs along the ilio-pubien branch, continues under the symphysis pubis and gives rise tot the arteries of the penial bulb, and the deep and dorsla arteries of the penis.

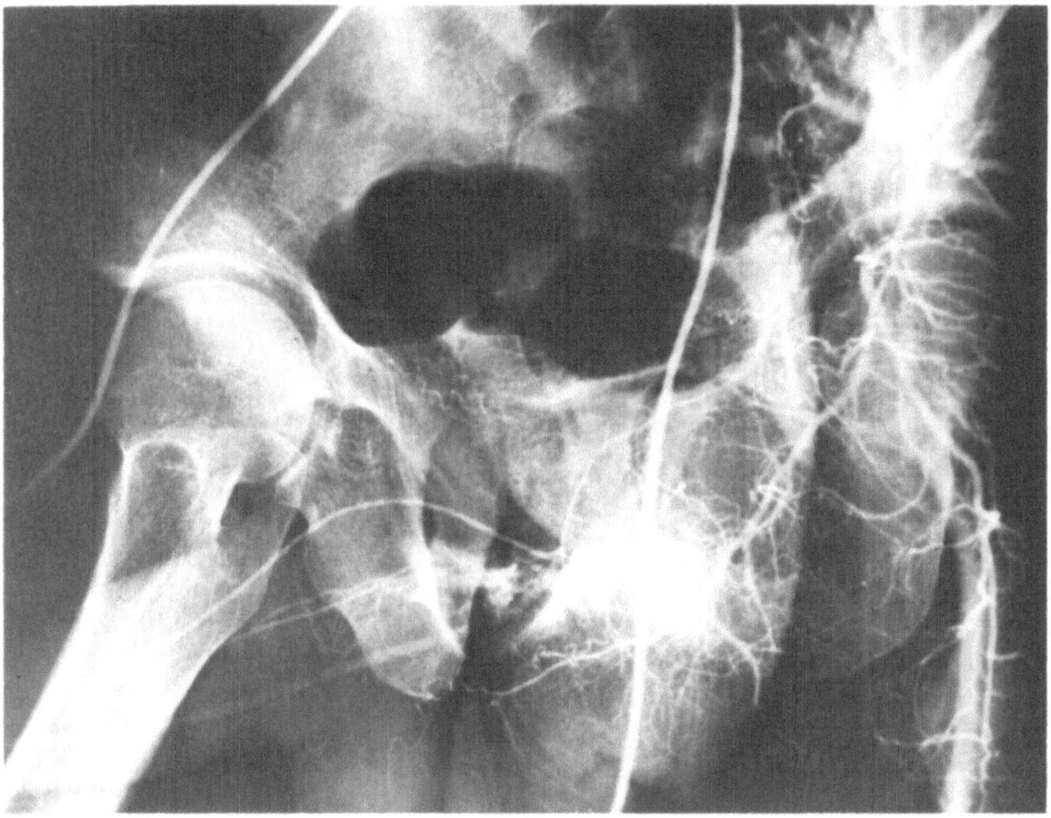

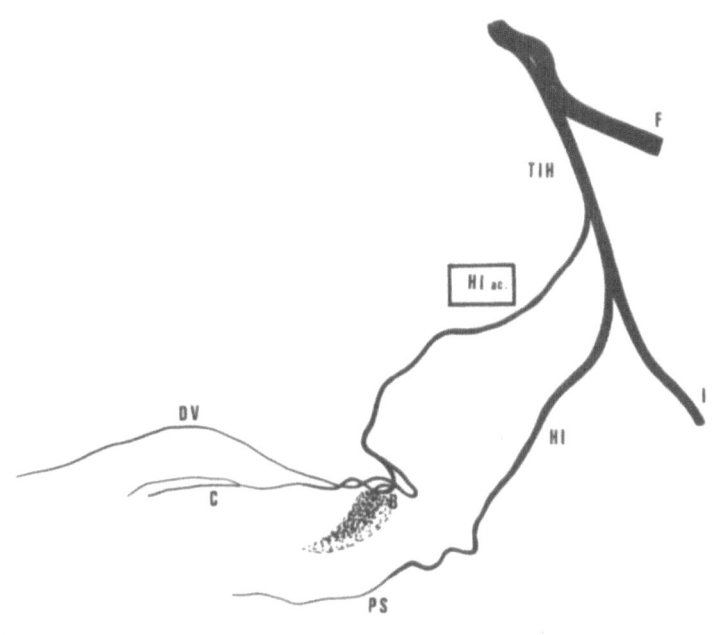

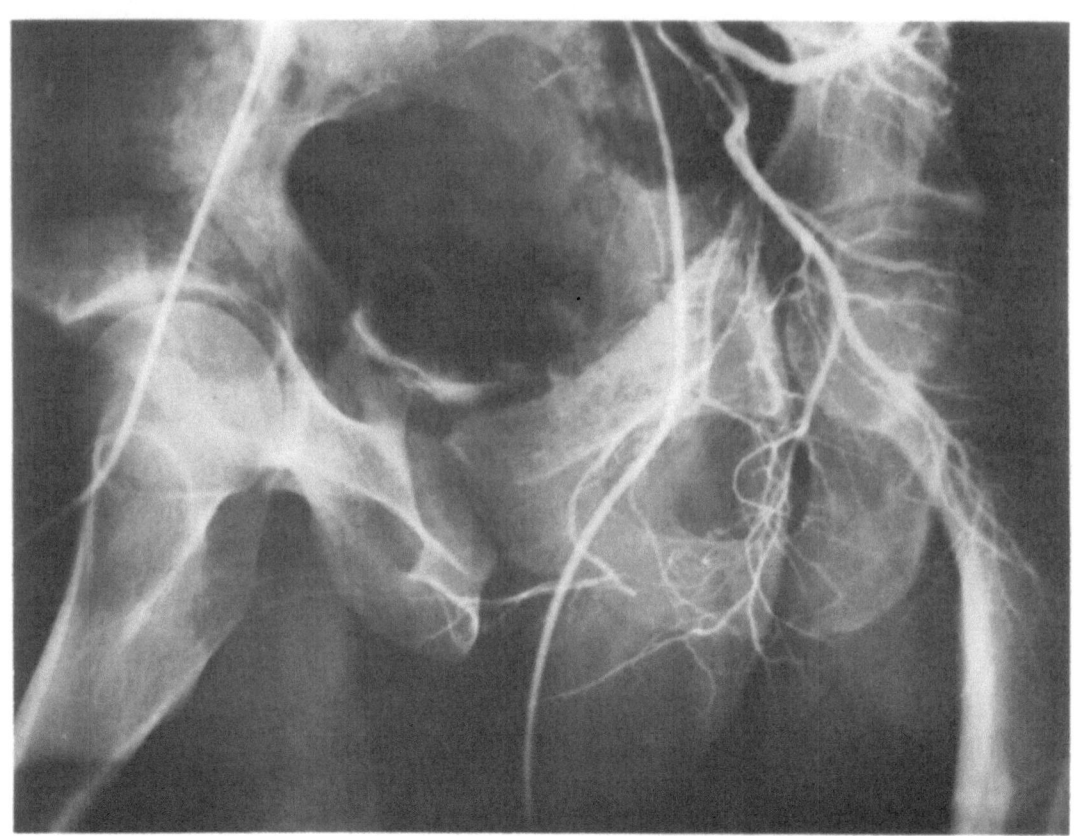

Fig. 27-28 - Antomy of internal pudendal artery

The superficial perineal artery is the terminal branch of the internal pudendal artery.

An accessory internal pudendal branch of the ischio-pudendal trunk descends the length of the ilio-pubien branch, turns around the anterior edge of the obturator foramen and after an anterior bend continues under the sub-pubien arch to give rise to the artery of the penial bulb, and the deep and dorsal arteries of the penis.

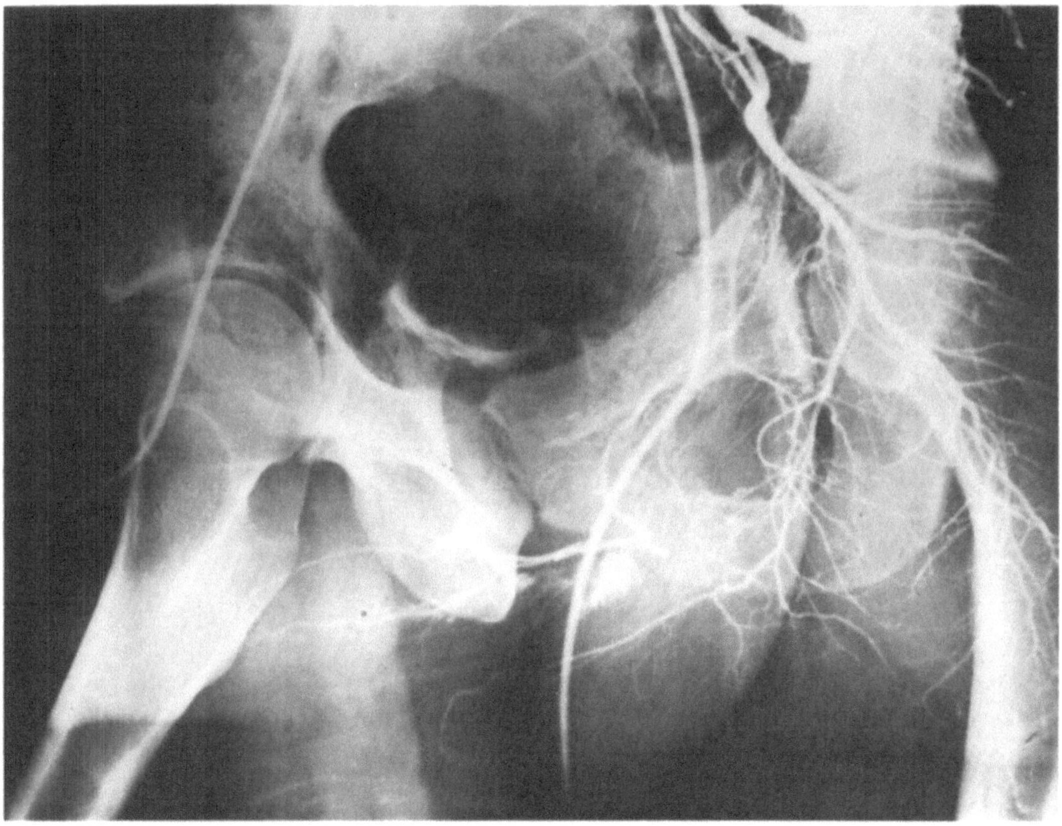

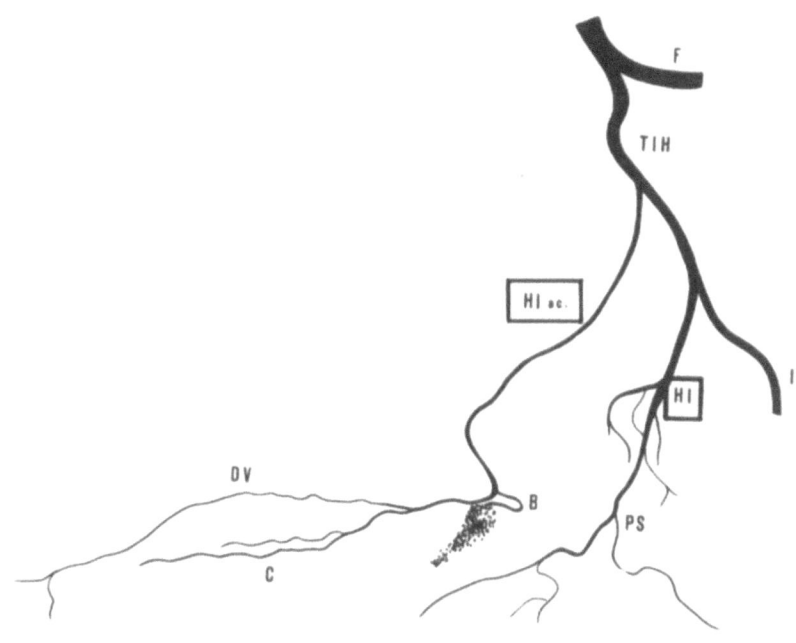

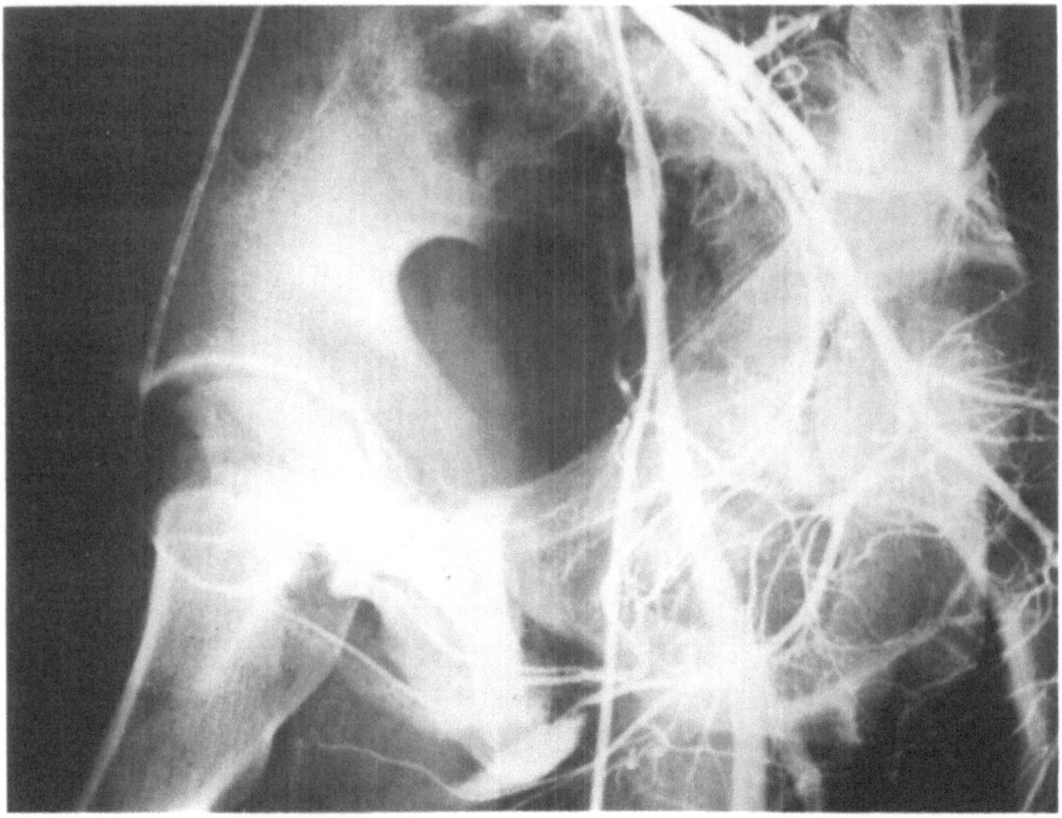

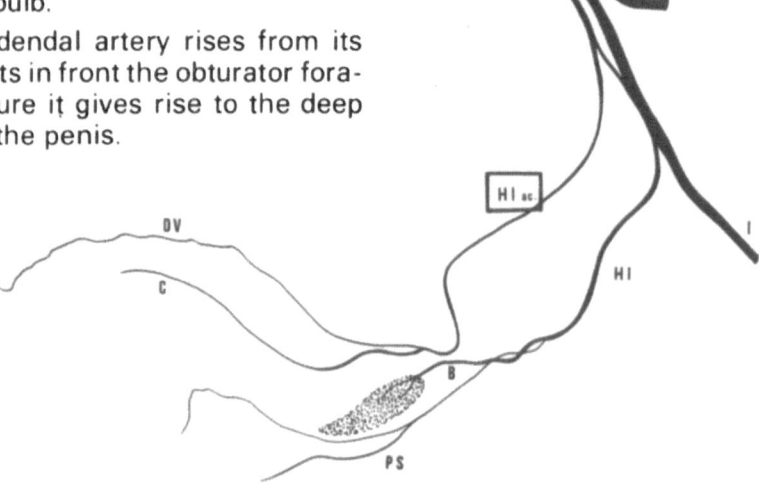

Fig. 29 - Accessory internal pudendal artery

Early division of ischio-pudendal trunk which is short.

Internal pudendal artery follows a normal course and terminates in giving the superficial perineal artery and artery of the bulb.

Accessory internal pudendal artery rises from its pelvic portion. It projects in front the obturator foramen, then after a flexure it gives rise to the deep and dorsal arteries of the penis.

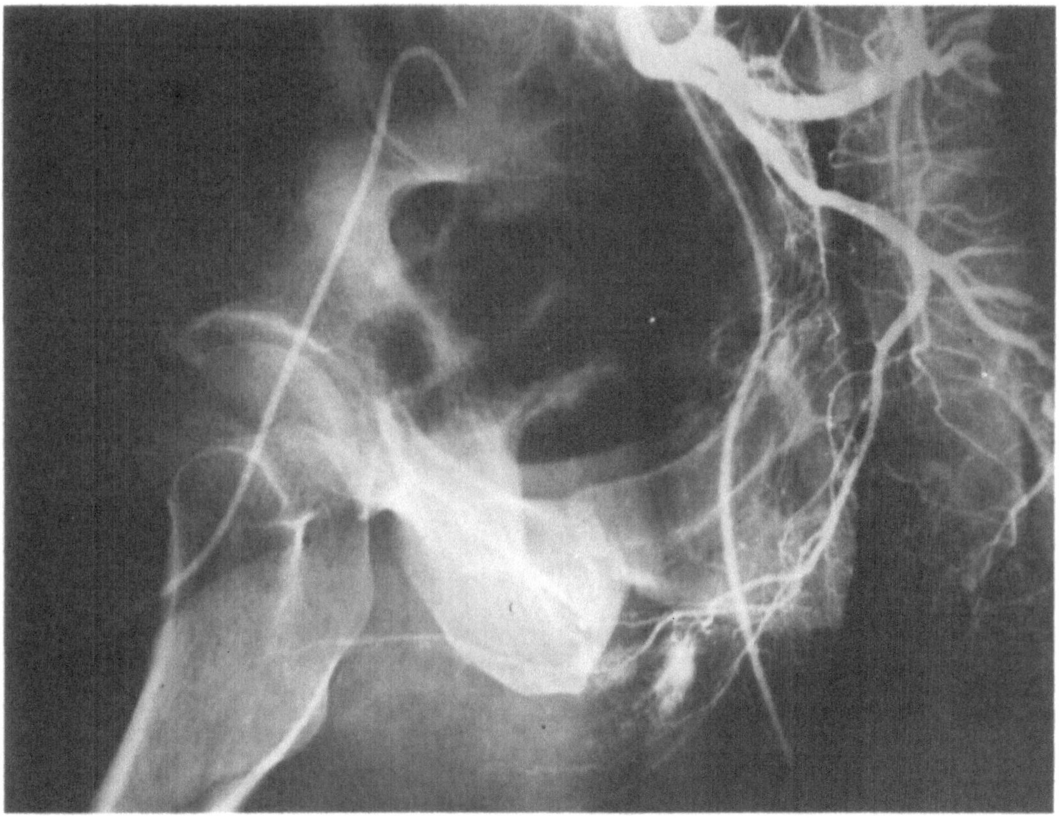

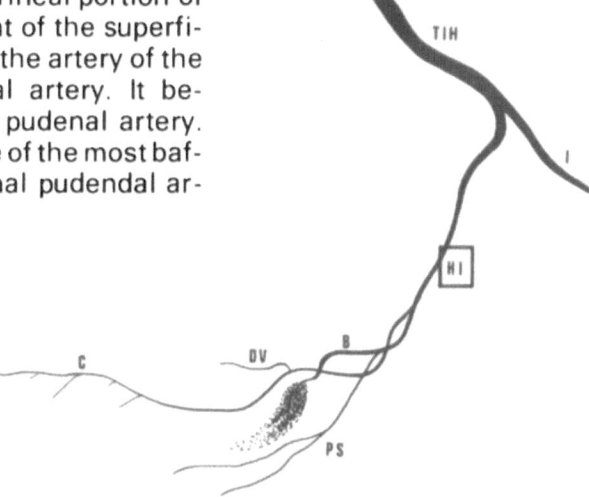

Fig. 30 - Anatomy of internal pudendal artery (variant)

The deep artery stems from the perineal portion of the internal pudendal artery in front of the superficial perineal artery and in this case the artery of the penial bulb becomes the terminal artery. It becomes a collateral of the internal pudenal artery. One can consider this aspect as one of the most baffling forms of the accessory internal pudendal artery.

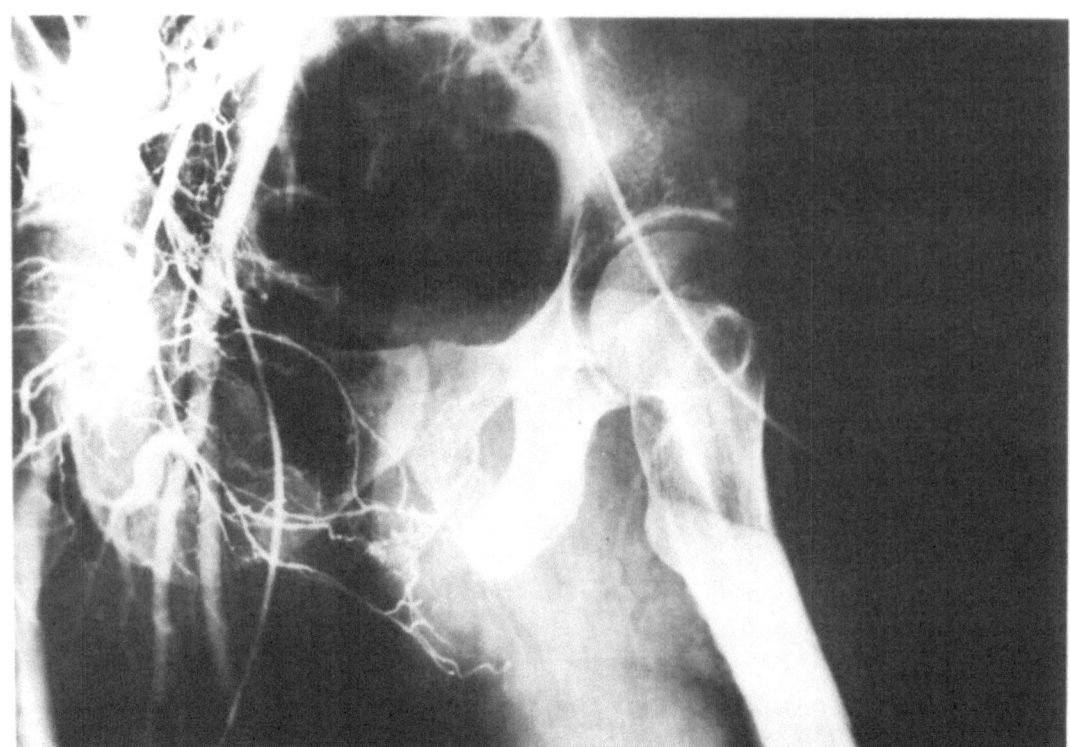

Fig. 31

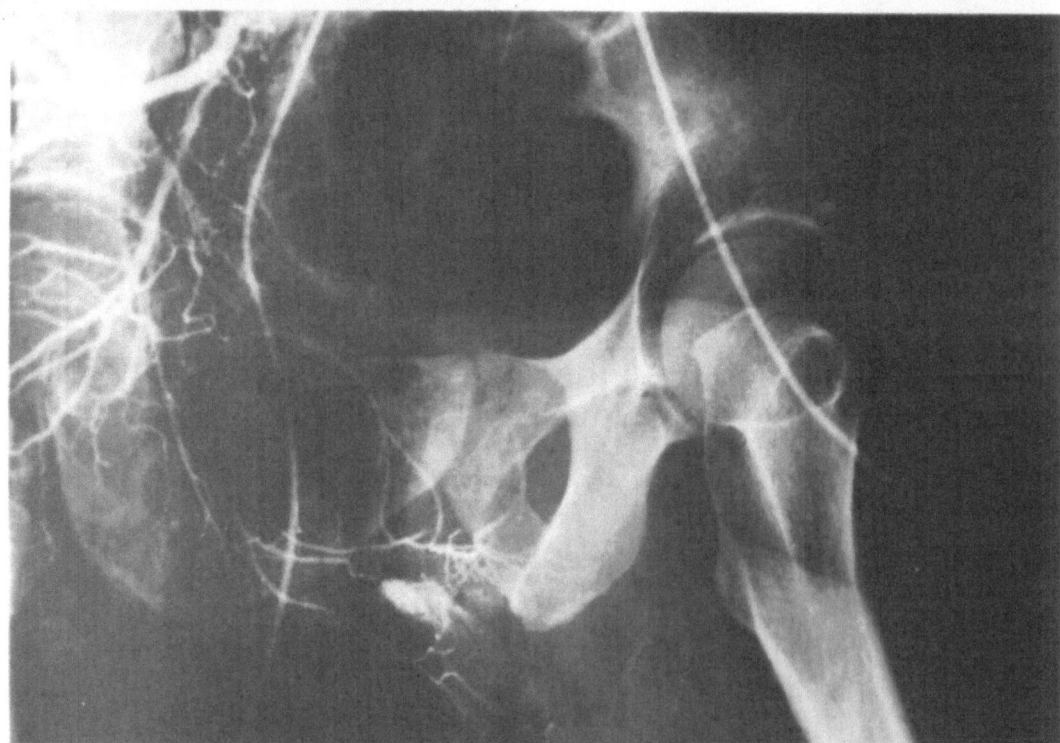

Fig. 32

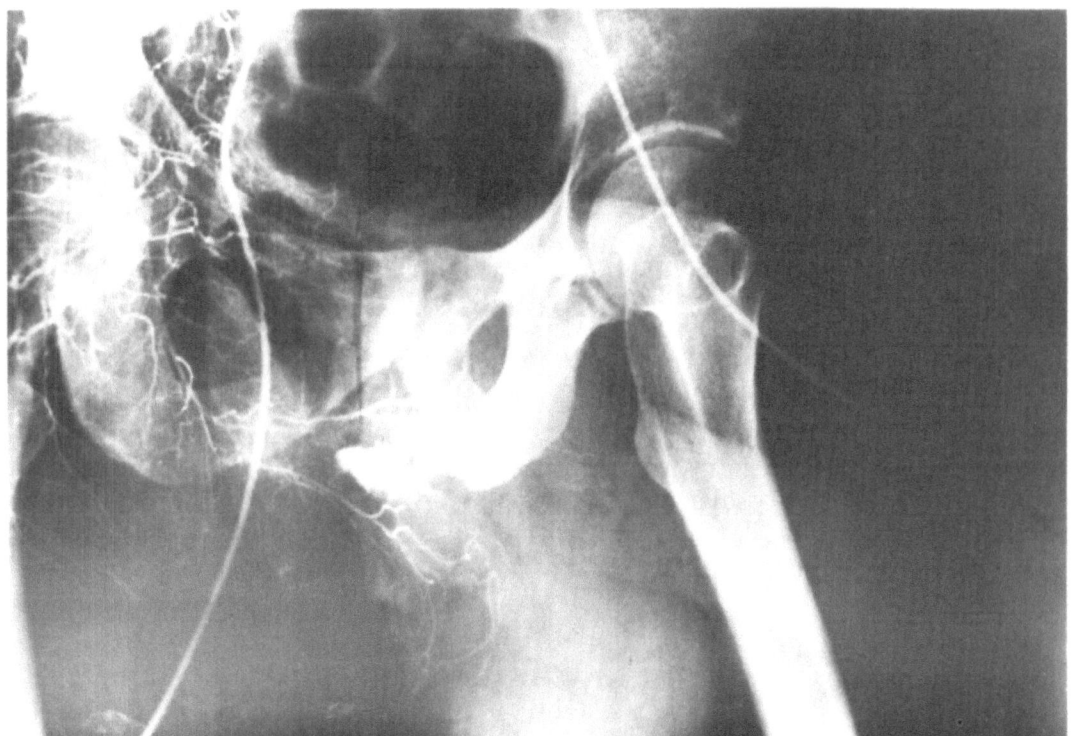

Fig. 33

Fig. 31-32-33 - Internal pudendal artery anastomosis with branch of hypogastric artery

Internal pudendal artery divides at level of inferior edge of obturator foramen in an inferior trunk superficial bulbo-perineal and a superior trunk which continues its normal direction up to the symphysis pubis.

Under symphysis pubis double anastomosis of internal pudendal artery with non systematisable artery which projects on ilio-pubien branch.

Amputation of dorsal artery of penis.

Atheromatous stenoses on deep artery which is of double composition. Only the posterior half is opacified.

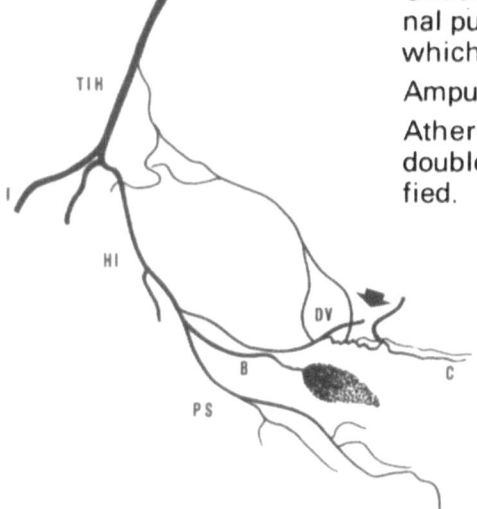

Terminal branches

● *Deep artery of the penis*

It arises in front of the artery of the penile bulb, has a straight course parallel to the axis of the penis and is projected above the urethra. Its posterior two thirds are always visible, its anterior third not always. There exists a late parenchymal, cavernous, stage of opacification involving the posterior two thirds of the organ, rarely the anterior third. In two cases we have noted the existence of two deep arteries for each corpus cavernosum.

● *Dorsal artery of the penis*

It reaches the upper border of the penis, travels along it as far as the base of the glans, and ends at the level of the arterial corona of the glans. In certain cases there is retrograde opacification of the dorsal artery on the opposite side, starting at the arterial corona. The branches of the dorsal artery are only occasionally visible. The lateral cavernous twigs are identified most frequently.

ACCESSORY INTERNAL PUDENDAL ARTERY

In six per cent of the cases we have observed the existence of an accessory internal pudendal artery (artery of Quain). It arises either from the internal pudendal artery, the internal iliac artery, or one of the latter's branches. Its course is different from that of the internal pudendal. It is projected above the obturator foramen, along the iliopubic ramus, descends along the pubis, turns posteriorly and reaches the pubic arch.

It gives origin to the deep and the dorsal arteries of the penis, sometimes also to the artery of the penile bulb.

ARTERIOGRAPHY OF INTERNAL PUDENDAL ARTERY

PATHOLOGIC RŒENTGEN ANATOMY

I) SYMPTOMATOLOGY

— Obstructions
— Dysplasies

II) DISTRIBUTION OF LESIONS

— Topographic distribution of obstructive lésions
— Topographic distribution of dysplasias
— Distribution of lésions according to
the degree of impotence
— Distribution of lesions according to age

III) ETIOLOGY

SYMPTOMATOLOGY

We have observed two types of arterial lesions : obstructions and dysplasias.

I) OBSTRUCTIONS

We shall not discuss obstructive lesions or severe stenoses of the aortic crossroads and the common iliac arteries.

The pathology of the crossroads is the real problem. Impotence is but one clinical sign among others. However, it should not be forgotten that it may be due to an associated lesion of an internal iliac or an internal pudendal artery.

Two consequences result. We must (1) direct the vascular surgeon toward operative techniques which do not jeopardize a possible secondary operation for impotence ; and (2) make a secondary arteriographic exploration of this impotence if it persists after the obstruction of the aortoiliac axes has been eliminated.

Lesions of the internal iliac artery

Amputations or pronounced stenoses of the internal iliac artery which are not associated with lesions developed from the common and external iliac are the exception. In those cases in which a lesion developed in the internal iliac artery, impotence is most of the time a symptom. In amputation of the internal iliac artery we have never observed a revascularization at a more distal level.

Lesions of the pelvic and gluteal portions of the internal pudendal artery

Atheromatous notches are present. Pronounced stenoses or amputations are exceptional. In these cases, we have not observed any distal revascularization.

Lesions of the ischiorectal portion of the internal pudendal artery

The signs are analogous to those of the two upper segments : atheromatous notches, pronounced stenoses and, exceptionally, amputations sometimes associated with distal revascularization.

Lesions of the perineal portion

Lesions of the internal pudendal artery occur most frequently in this portion : pronounced stenoses and amputations. Pictures of occlusion are sometimes associated with distal revascularizations.

Lesions of the deep and dorsal arteries of the penis

Besides atheromatous notches which give to these arteries the appearance of wires, we find here stenoses or amputations. There is no downstream revascularization.

II) DYSPLASIAS

Only nine cases of dysplasia have been observed. The clinical picture is characteristic. There is incomplete erection associated with deviation of the penis to the affected side in a patient who never had a normal erection.

Four types of rœntgenographies were noted.

— unilateral hypotrophy of the penile arteries (deep and dorsal arteries of penis and artery of the bulb) ;

— hypotrophy of one accessory internal pudendal artery and of the corresponding deep and dorsal arteries ;

— agenesis of one or more penile arteries ;

— agenesis of one or more penile arteries with compensatory hypertrophy of the contralateral vascular axes.

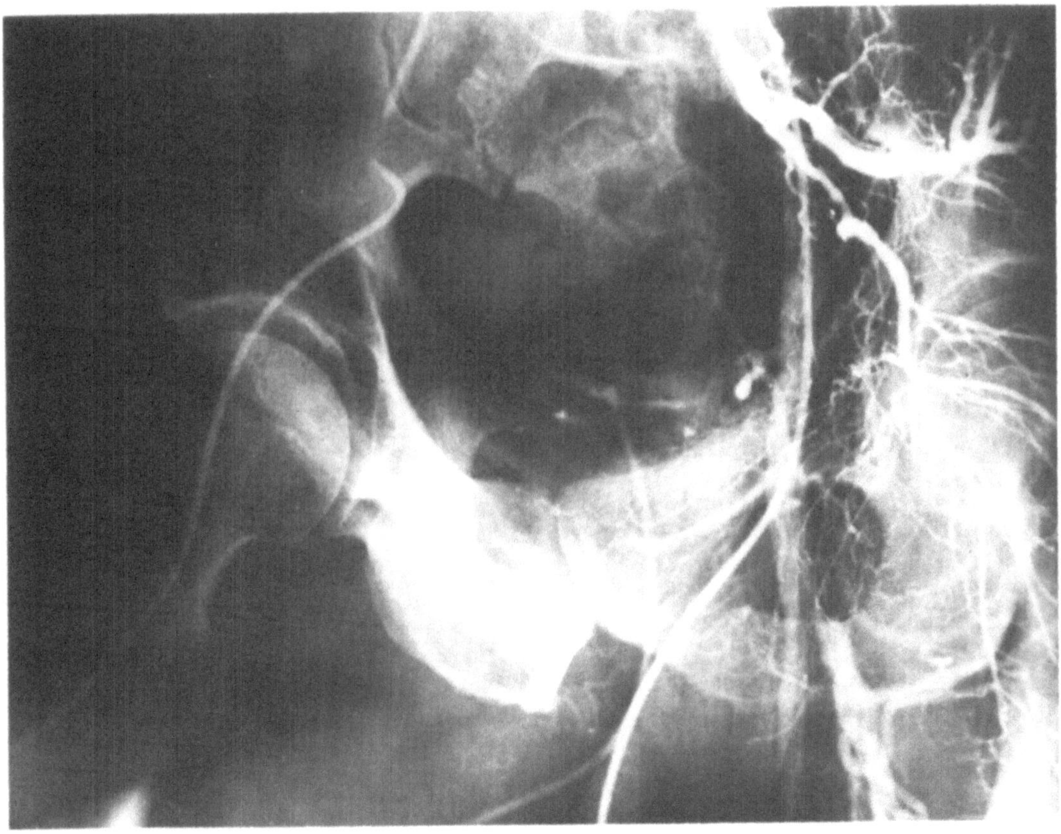

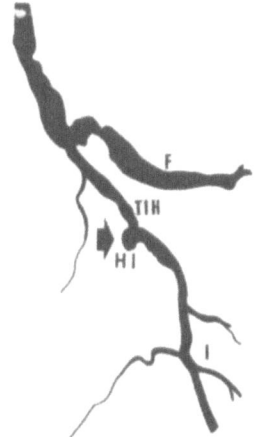

Fig. 34 - Amputation of internal pudendal artery

Atheromatous notches and stenoses at hypogastric artery level, gluteal artery level and ischio-pudendal trunk level.

Amputation of internal pudendal artery at origin.

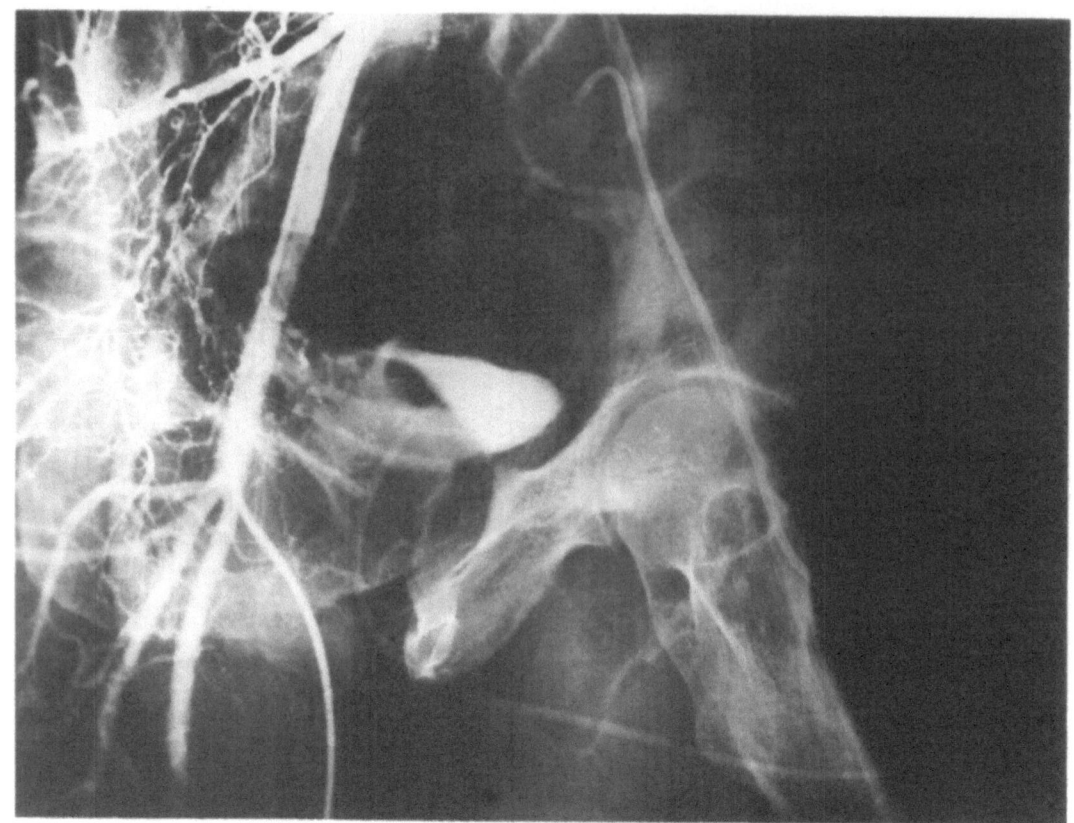

Fig. 35-36 - Amputation of ischio-pudendal trunk

Very thin aspect then amputated from ischio-pudendal trunk.

Partial reinjection of ischiatic artery by network of collaterals.

No opacification of internal pudendal artery.

Aortography shows rigidity of origin of primitive iliac artery and stenosis of origin of right renal artery. This was confirmed by selective renal arteriography.

Proximal lesions always are associated with diffused atheromatous lesions.

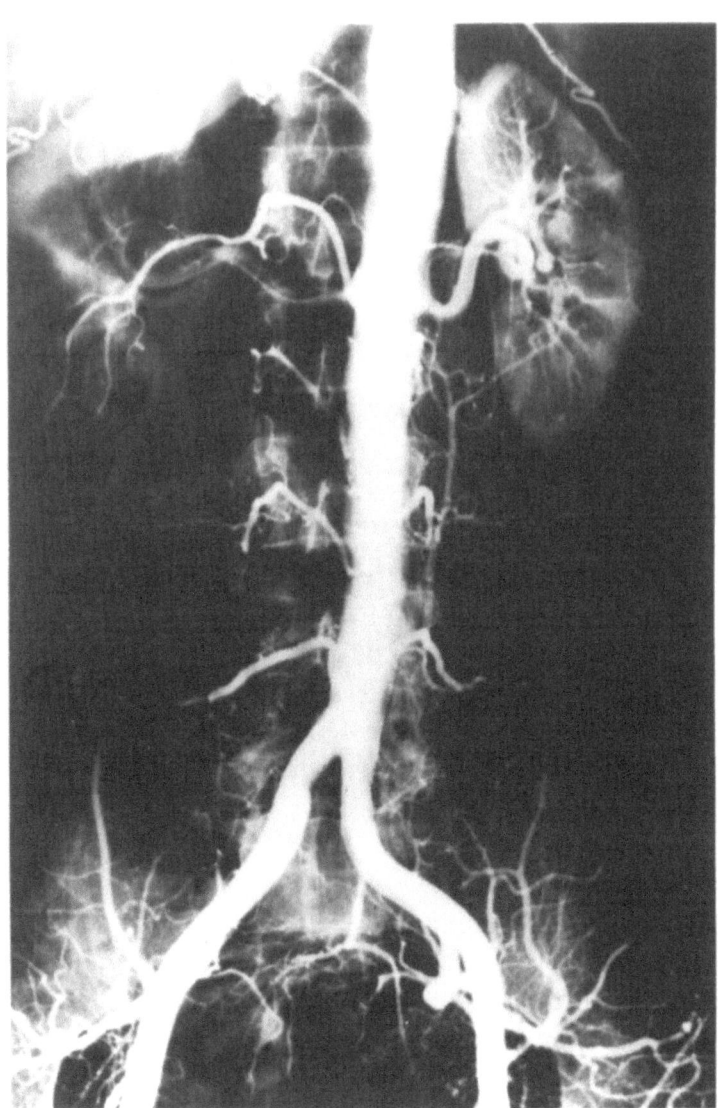

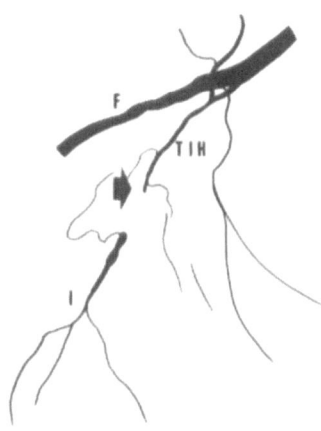

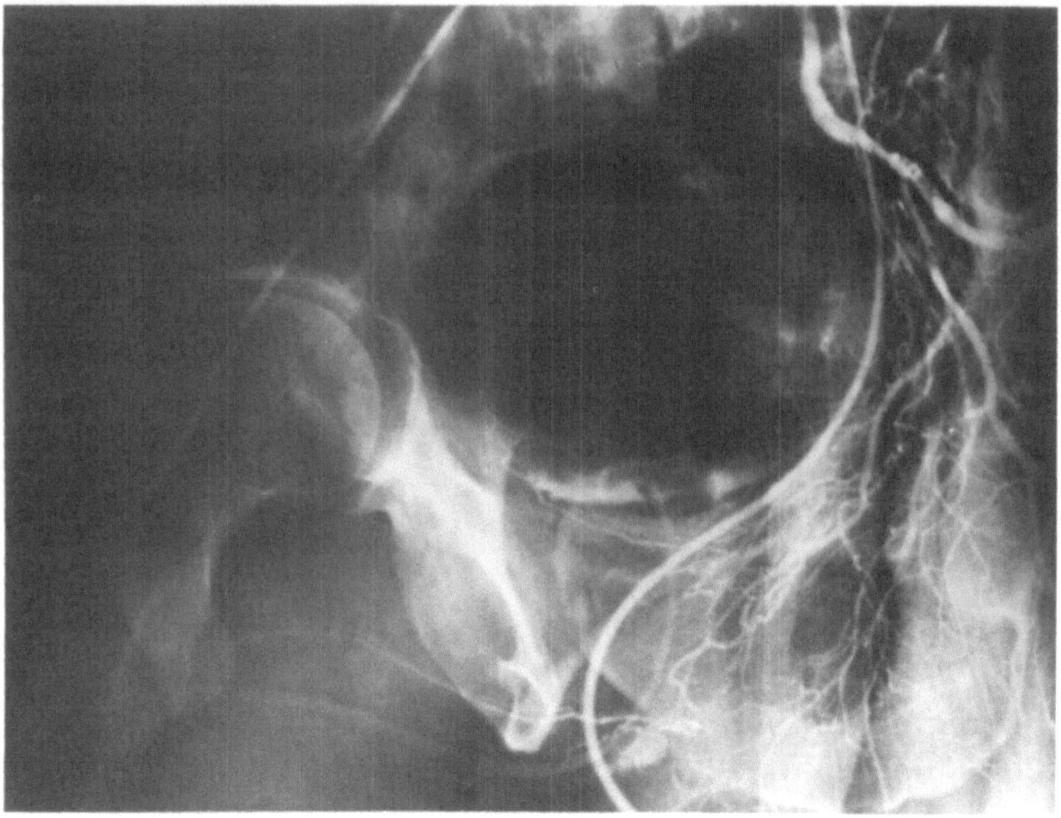

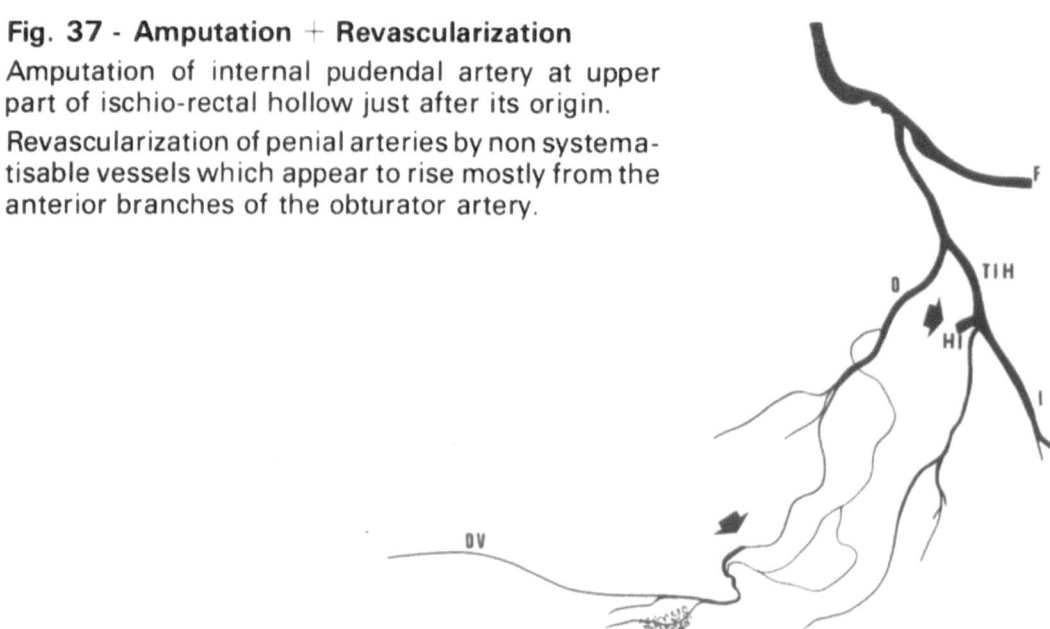

Fig. 37 - Amputation + Revascularization

Amputation of internal pudendal artery at upper part of ischio-rectal hollow just after its origin.

Revascularization of penial arteries by non systematisable vessels which appear to rise mostly from the anterior branches of the obturator artery.

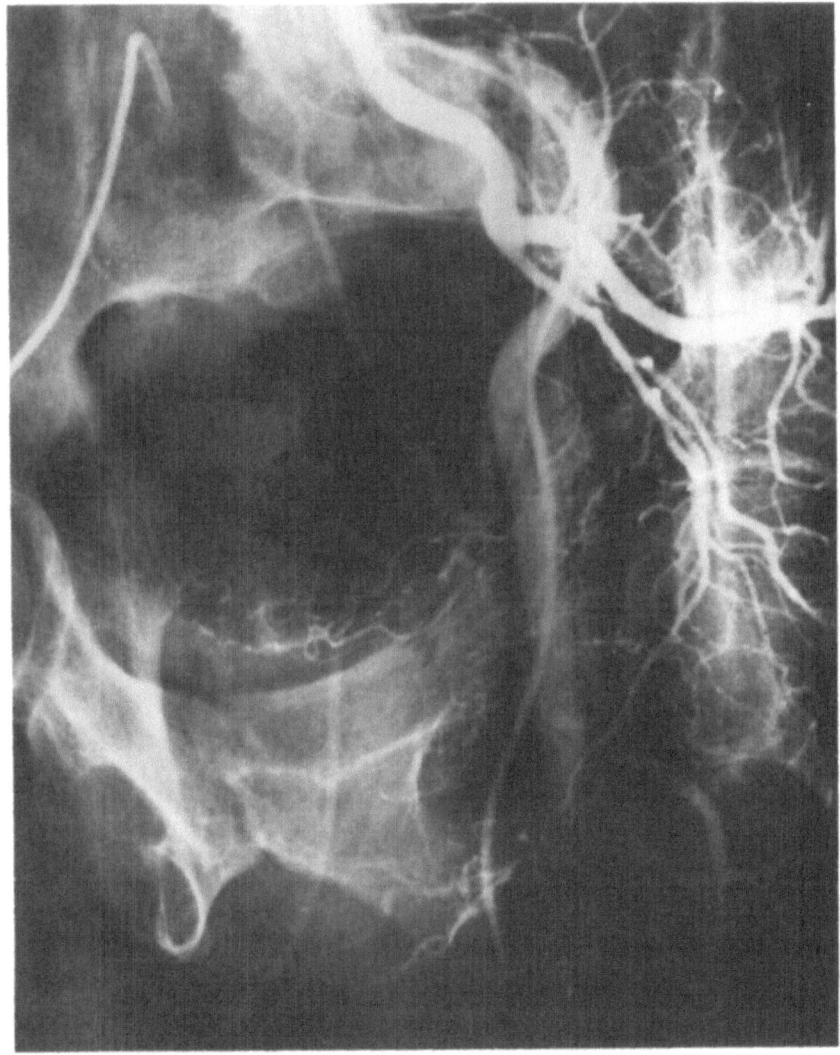

Fig. 38 - Amputation + revascularization

Amputation of internal pudendal artery at lower part of ischio-rectal segment.

Repermeabilization of origin of perineal portion of internal pudendal artery which is again amputated after the origin of superficial perineal artery.

HI

I

PS

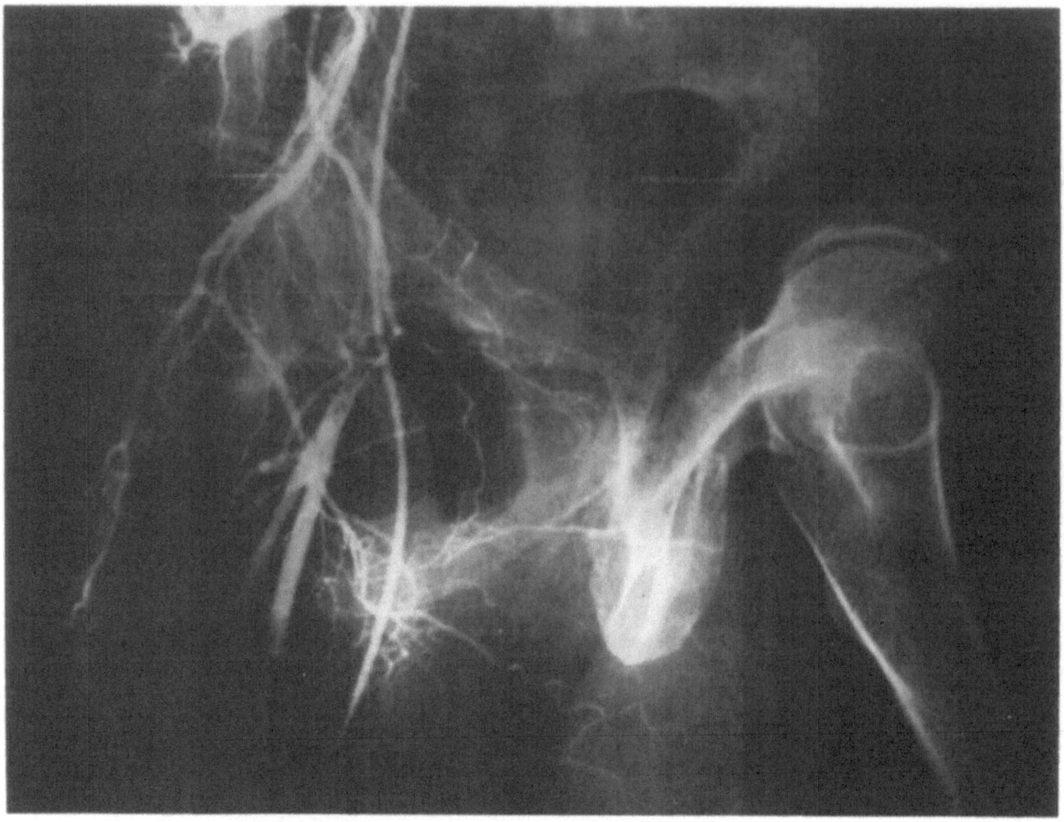

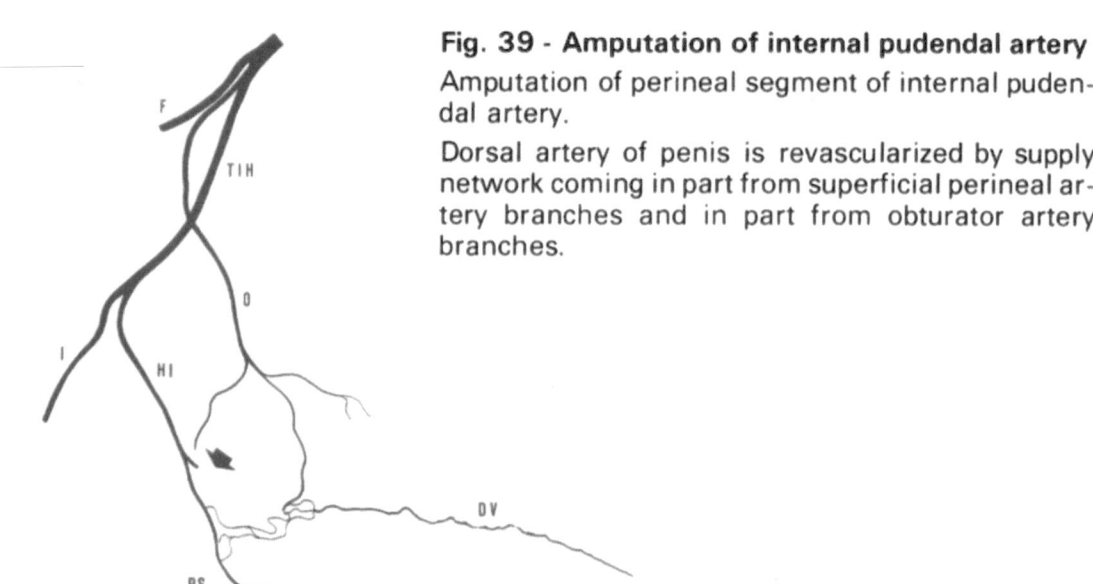

Fig. 39 - Amputation of internal pudendal artery

Amputation of perineal segment of internal pudendal artery.

Dorsal artery of penis is revascularized by supply network coming in part from superficial perineal artery branches and in part from obturator artery branches.

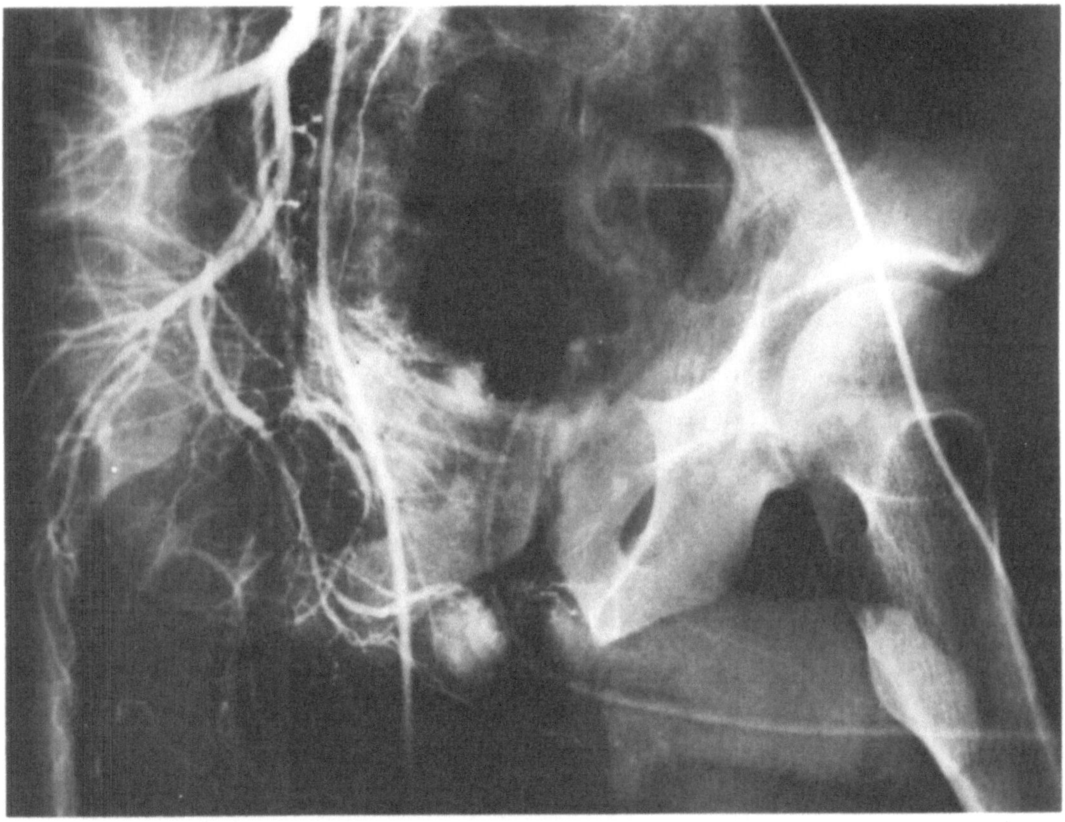

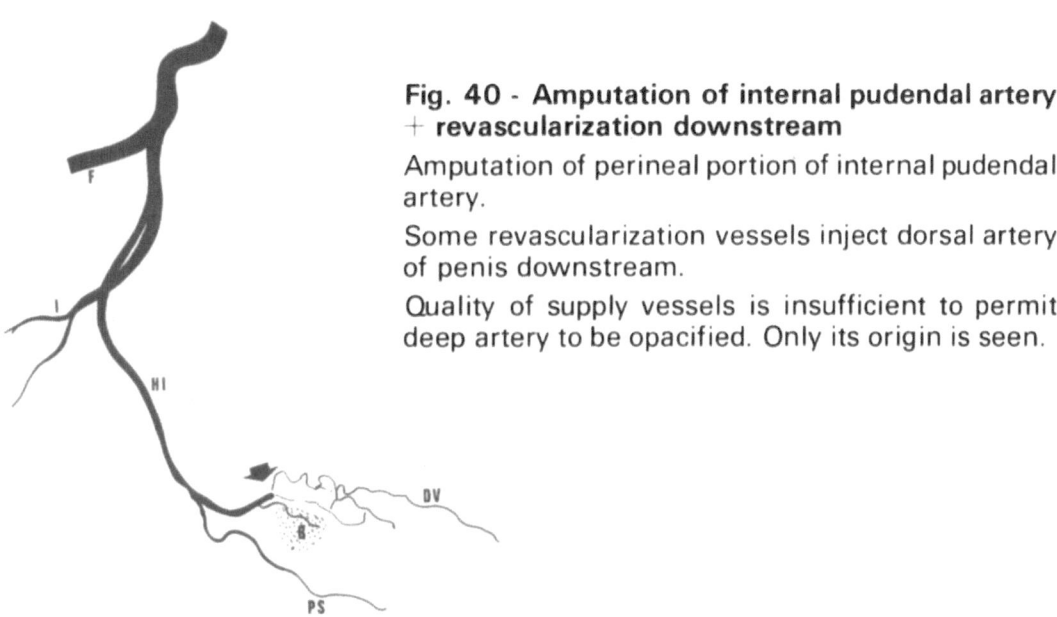

Fig. 40 - Amputation of internal pudendal artery + revascularization downstream

Amputation of perineal portion of internal pudendal artery.

Some revascularization vessels inject dorsal artery of penis downstream.

Quality of supply vessels is insufficient to permit deep artery to be opacified. Only its origin is seen.

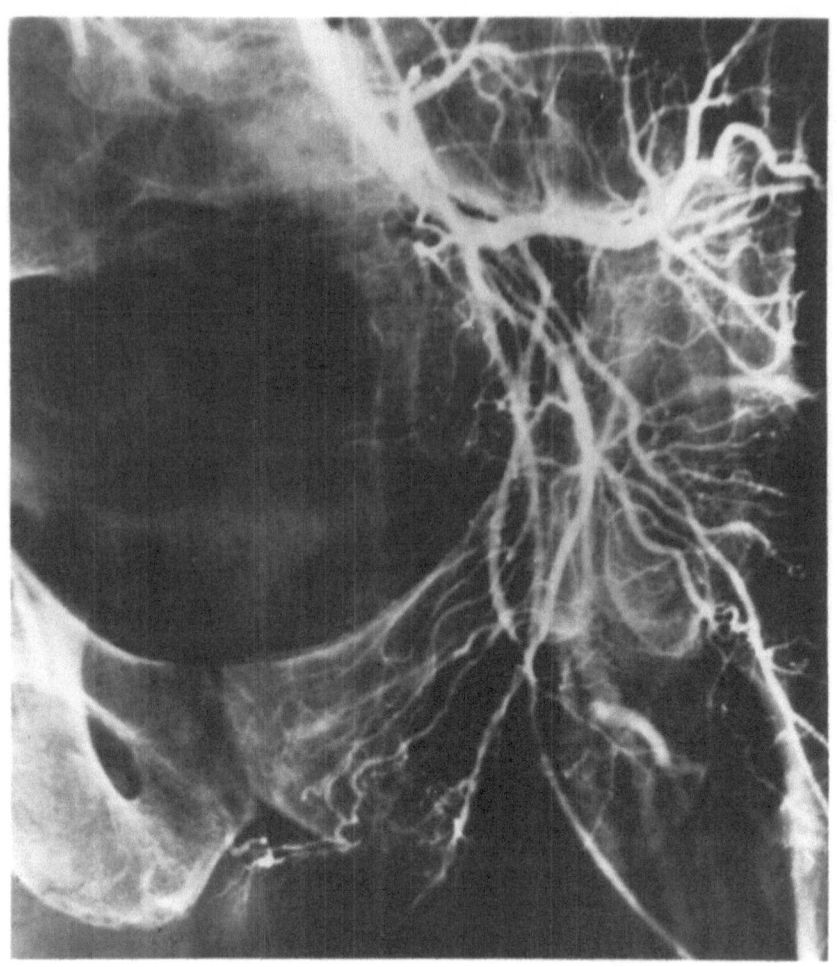

Fig. 41-42 - Amputation + revascularization

Internal pudendal artery is amputated just after origin of superficial perineal artery.

Supply vessels revascularize dorsal artery of penis which shows some atheromatous stenoses at its proximal third level. Deep artery also revascularized in same manner and also shows some atheromatous stenoses at proximal third level, then it is very thin.

Artery of penial bulb is excluded.

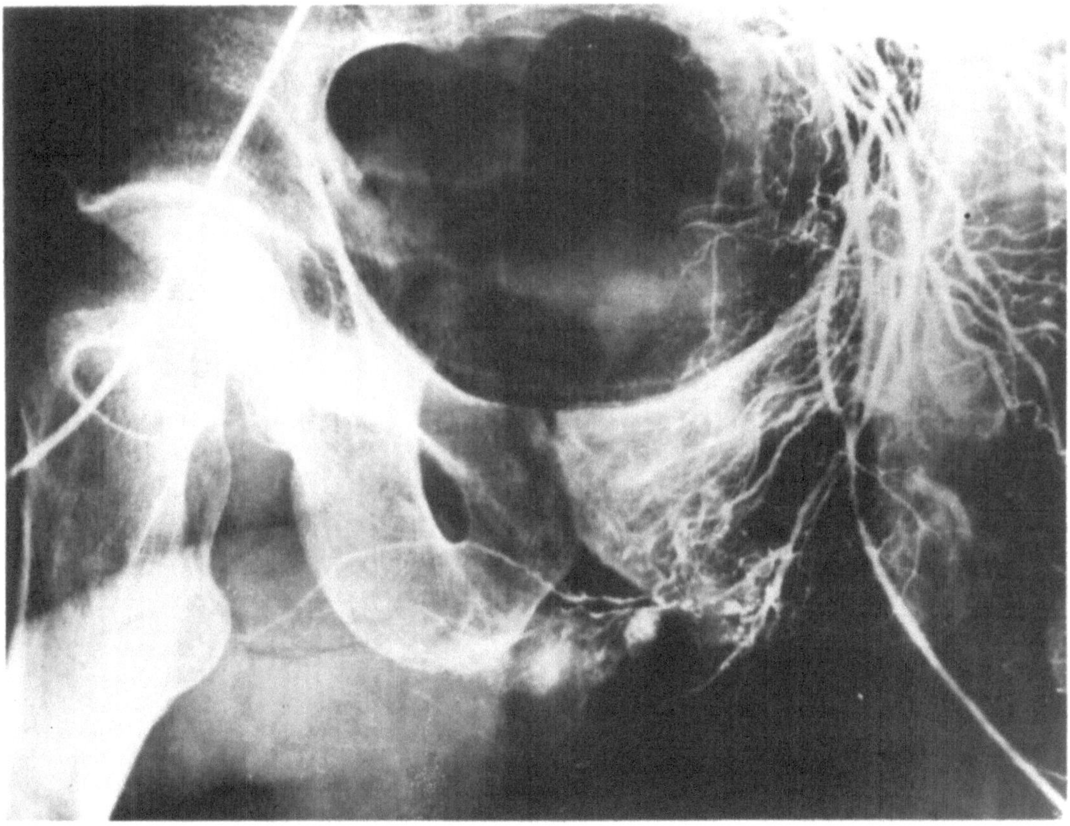

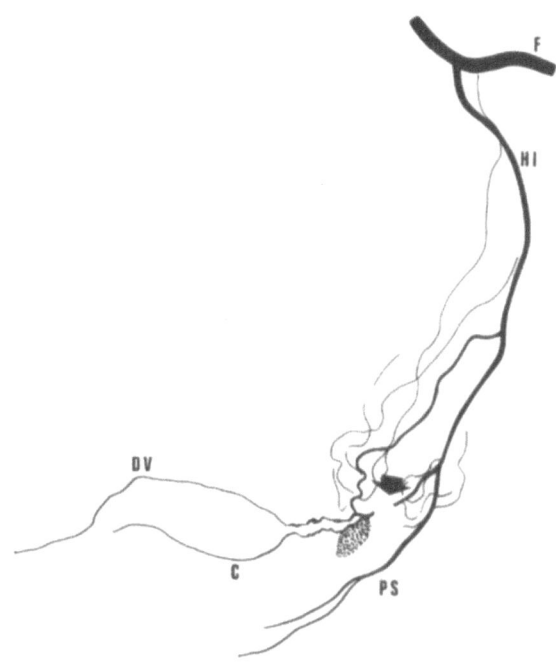

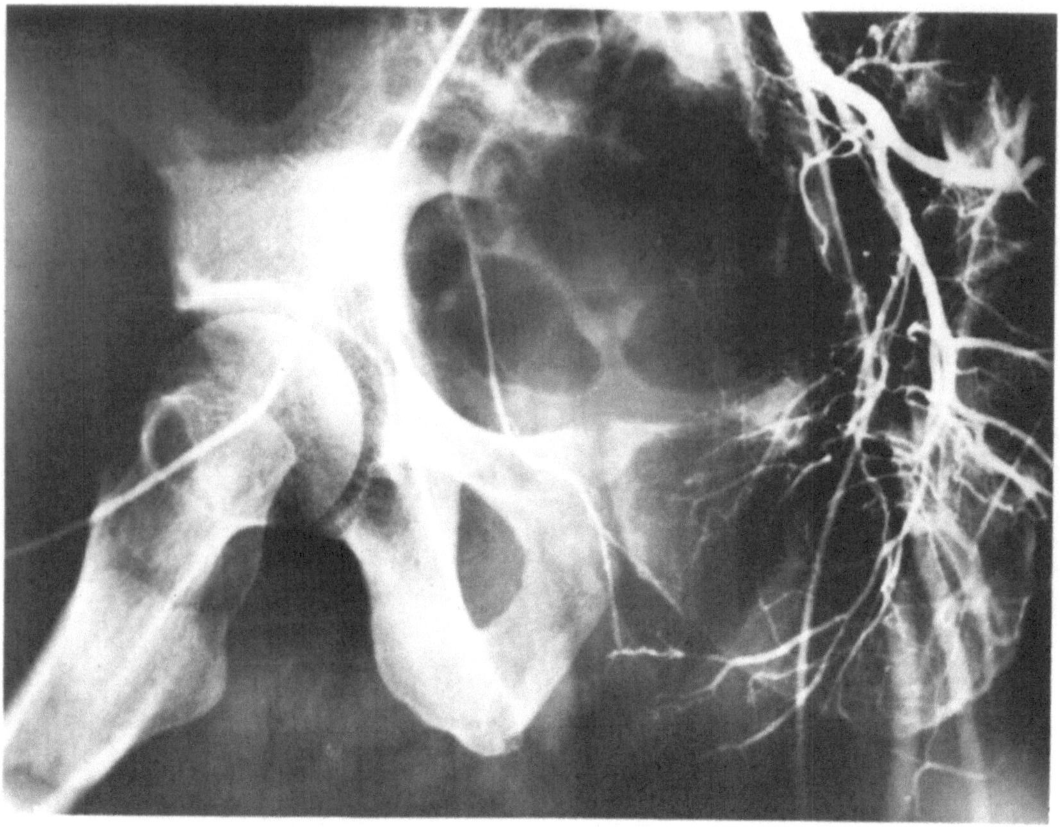

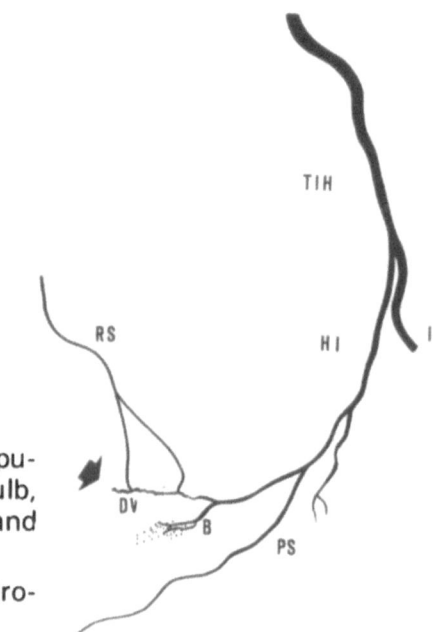

Fig. 43 - Stenoses + Amputation

Stenoses at level of terminal portion of internal pudendal artery after origin of artery of penial bulb, then amputation before origin of deep artery and dorsal artery of penis.

Because of this amputation, opacification of retrosymphysic artery is particularly dense.

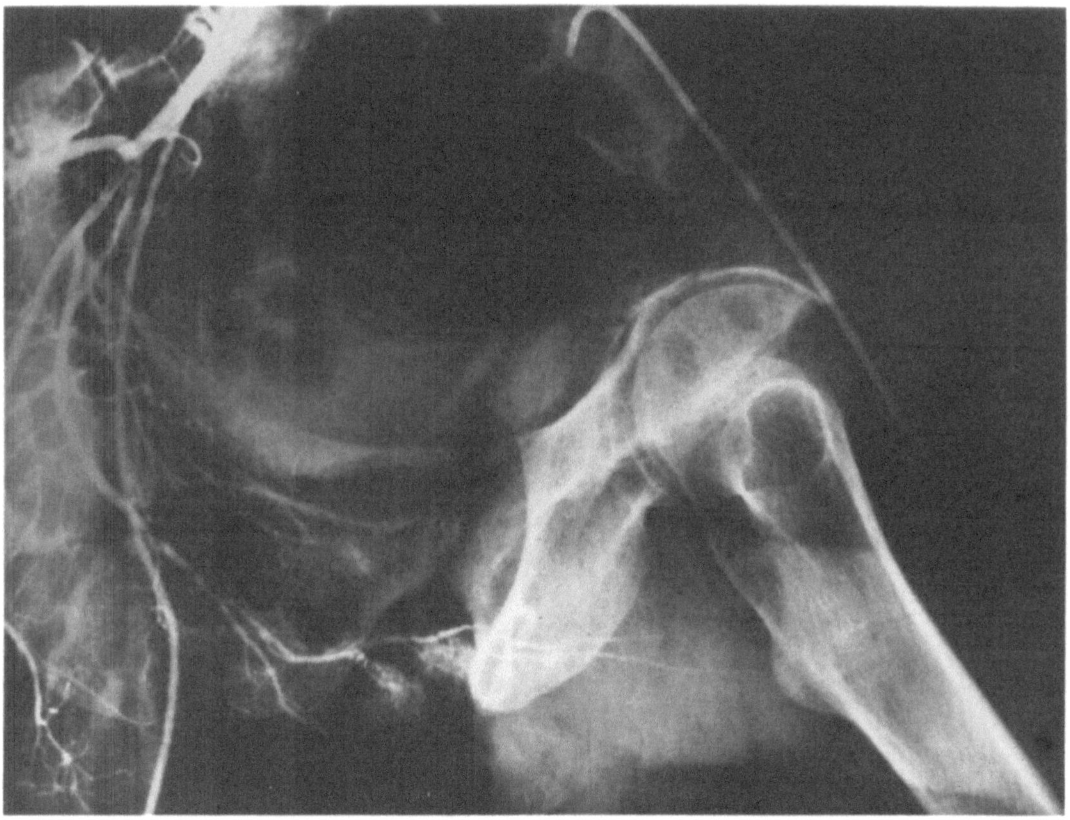

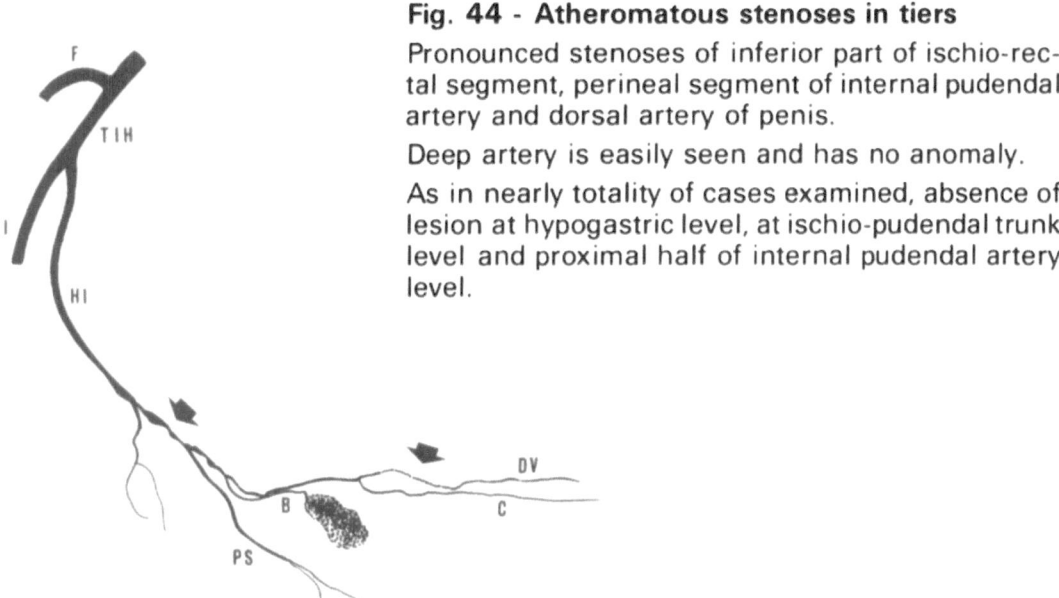

Fig. 44 - Atheromatous stenoses in tiers

Pronounced stenoses of inferior part of ischio-rectal segment, perineal segment of internal pudendal artery and dorsal artery of penis.

Deep artery is easily seen and has no anomaly.

As in nearly totality of cases examined, absence of lesion at hypogastric level, at ischio-pudendal trunk level and proximal half of internal pudendal artery level.

arteriography of internal pudendal artery/77

DISTRIBUTION OF LESIONS

I) TOPOGRAPHIC DISTRIBUTION OF OBSTRUCTIVE LESIONS

There are two large types of lesions :

Lesions of the internal iliac artery

Most often associated with lesions evolved from the common and external iliac arteries. They are part of the pathology of the iliac vessels.

Lesions of distal arteries

i.e. perineal portion of the internal pudendal artery, and deep and dorsal arteries of the penis. These are the most frequent causes of impotence of vascular origin.

II) TOPOGRAPHIC DISTRIBUTION OF DYSPLASIAS

We have observed these lesions only in penile arteries. All cases were unilateral.

In several patients we found narrowing of the entire internal pudendal axis. We did not register these cases as dysplasias, since our hemodynamic tests are not as yet precise enough to allow such assurance.

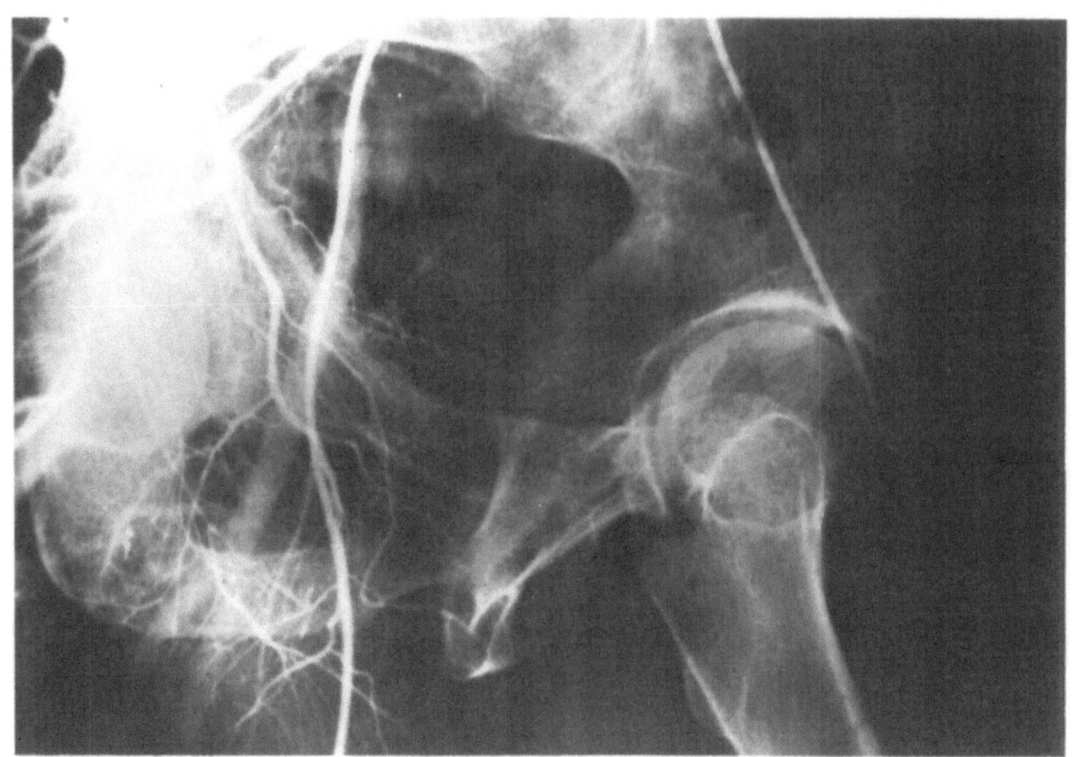

Fig. 45-46 - Vascular stenoses

Very thin aspect of ischio-recal portion and of perineal portion of internal pudendal artery. It is the base of numerous atheromatous notches in tiers.

Internal pudendal artery gives the artery of the penial bulb which is pathologic and dorsal artery of the penis.

An accessory internal pudendal artery, branch of the obturator artery gives the deep artery which is thin and amputated at its middle third level.

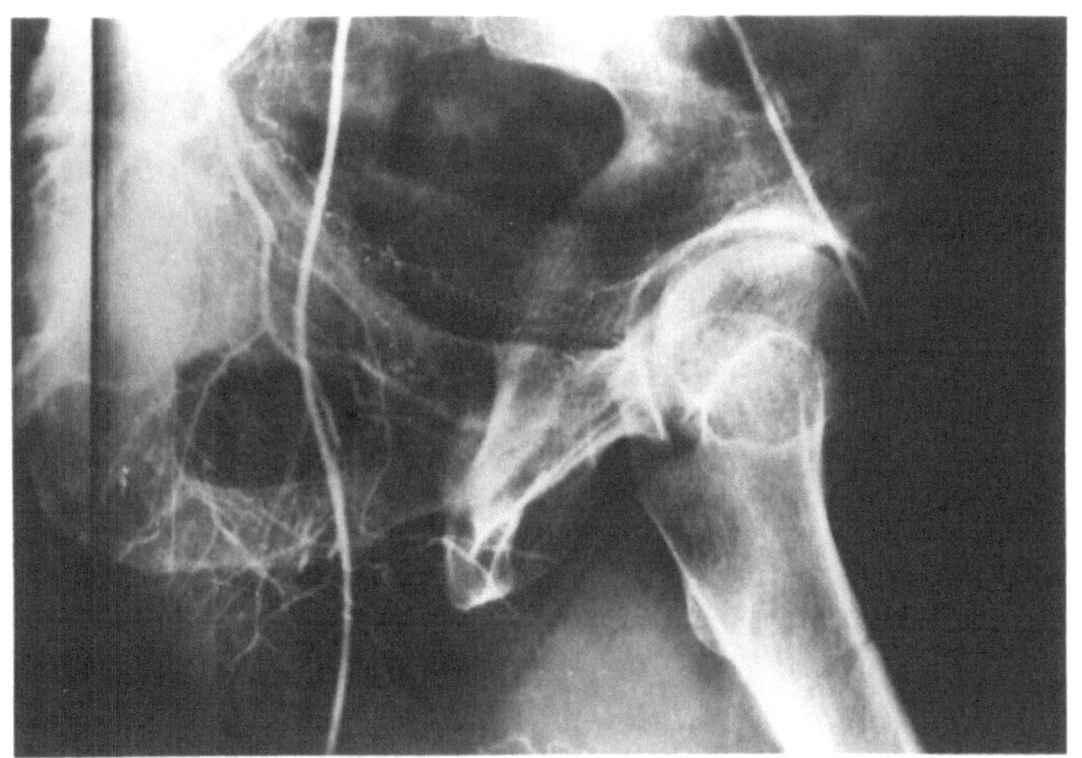

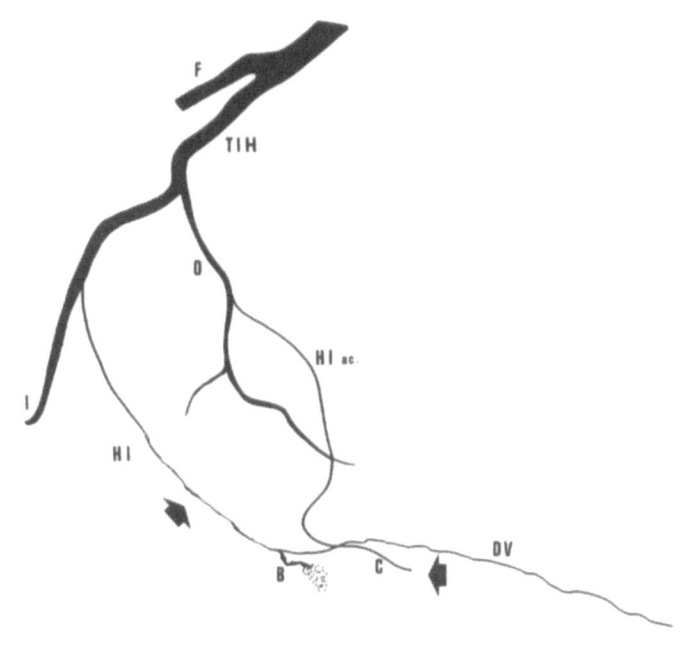

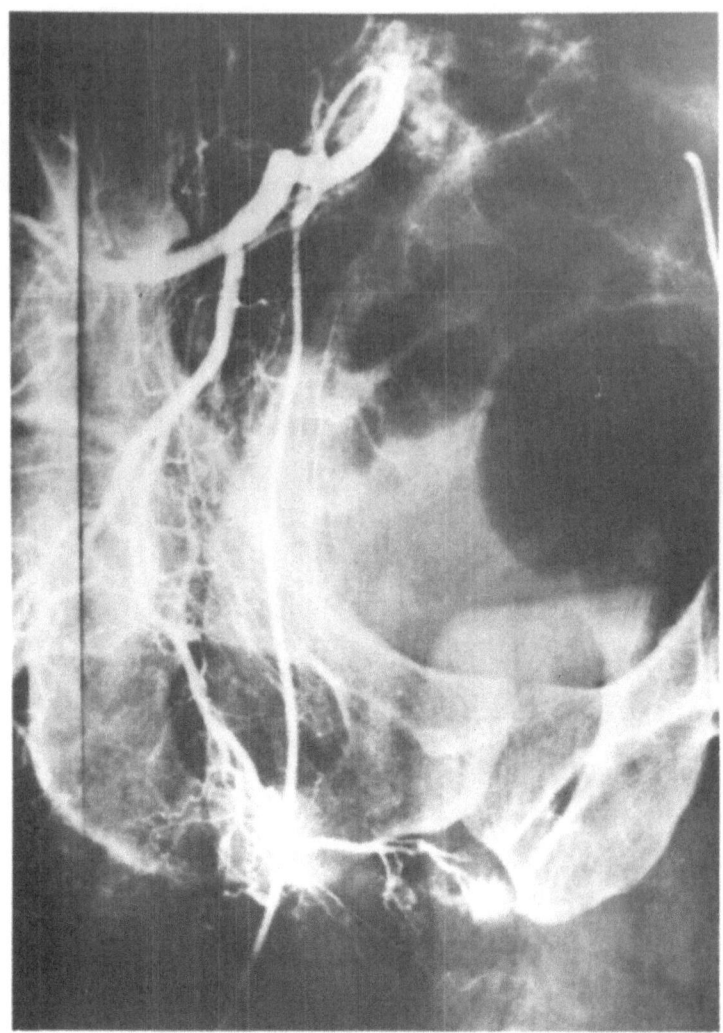

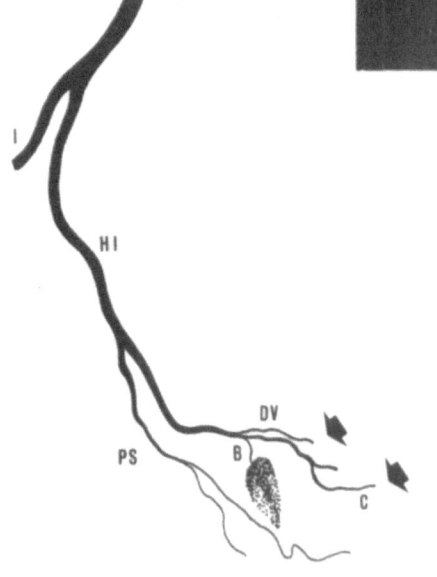

Fig. 47 - Amputation of deep artery and dorsal artery of penis

Dorsal artery of penis is amputated just after its origin.

Only posterior portion of deep artery is opacified. Its anterior 3/4 are excluded.

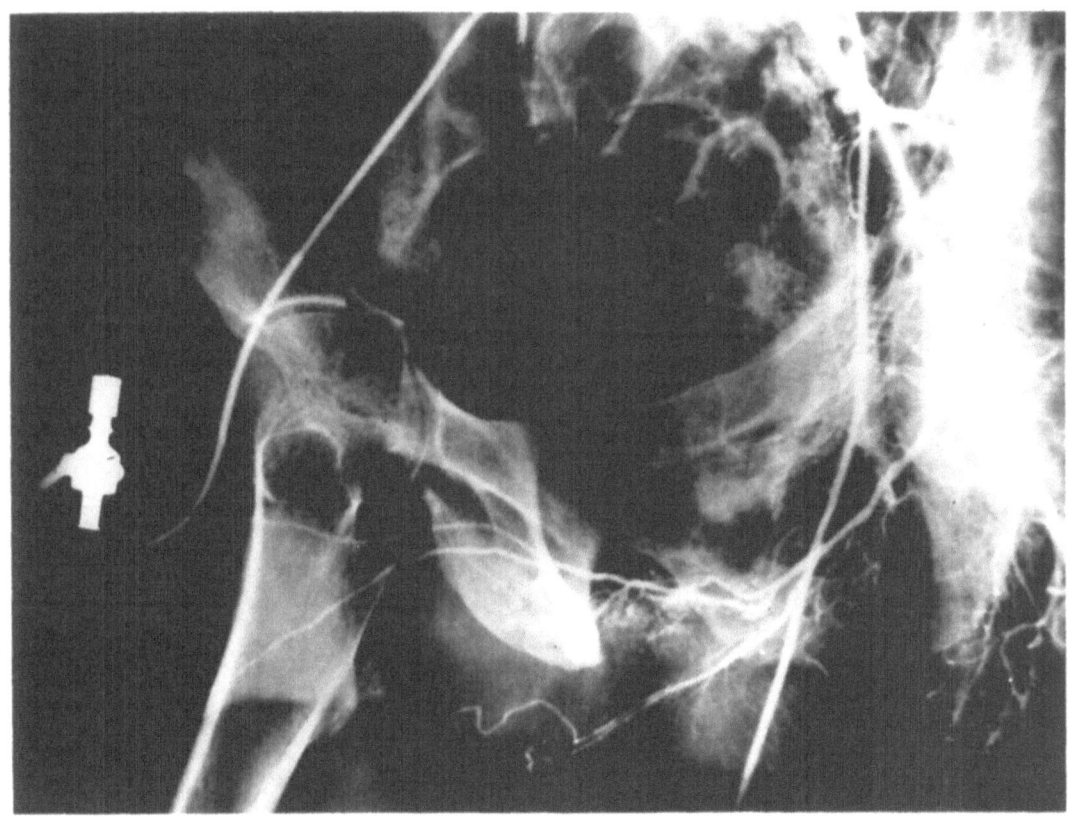

Fig. 48 - Atheromatous stenoses + amputation

Atheromatous stenoses of terminal portion of internal pudendal artery (after origin of artery of penial bulb).

Amputation of deep artery just after its origin.

Voluminous ramus of dorsal of penis for teguments.

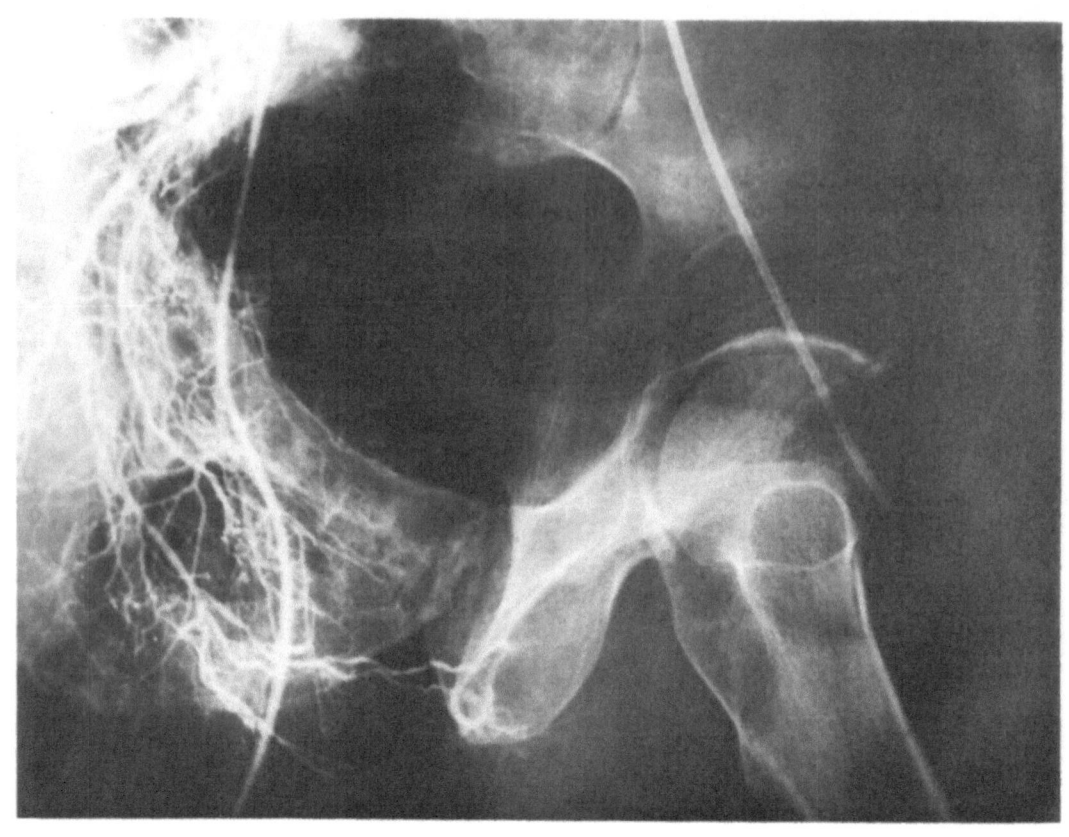

Fig. 49-50 - Stenoses + amputation

Pronounced stenosis of perineal portion of internal pudendal artery after origin of perineal artery.

Amputation of deep artery at junction third posterior - third medium.

84/*radiologic exploration of impotence*

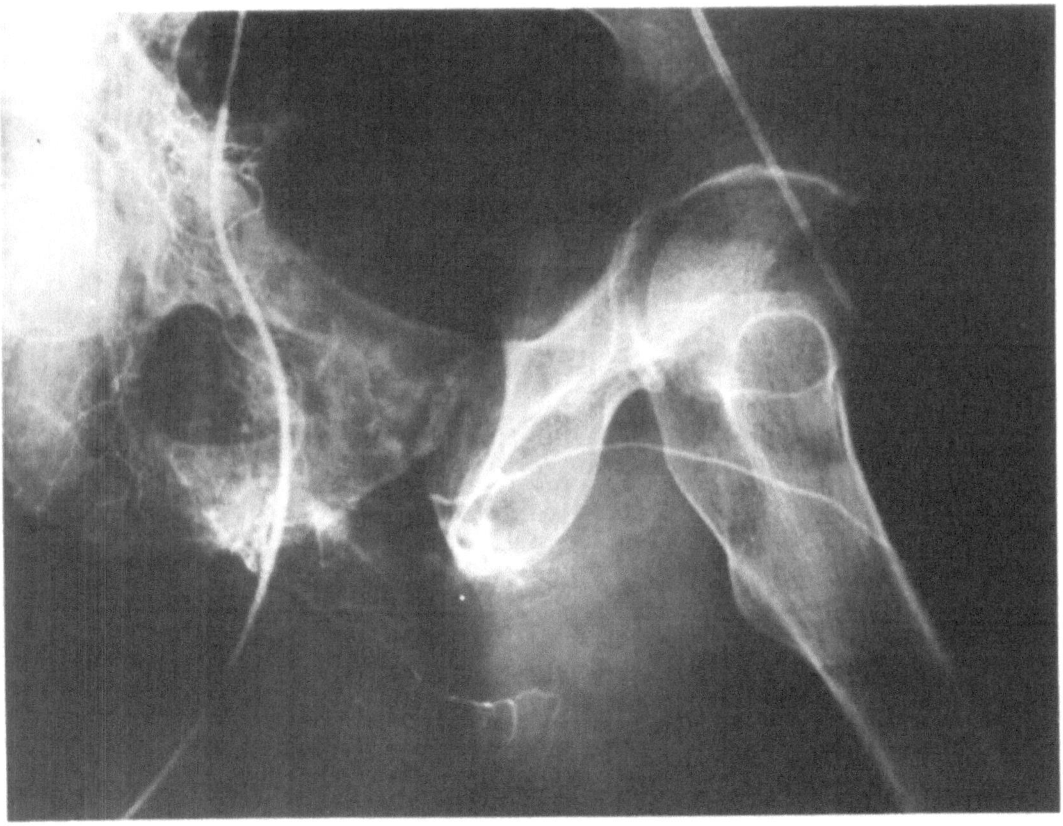

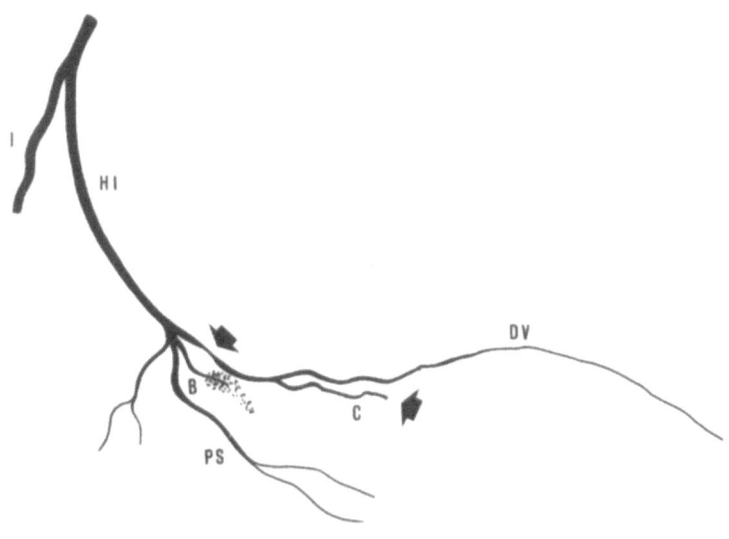

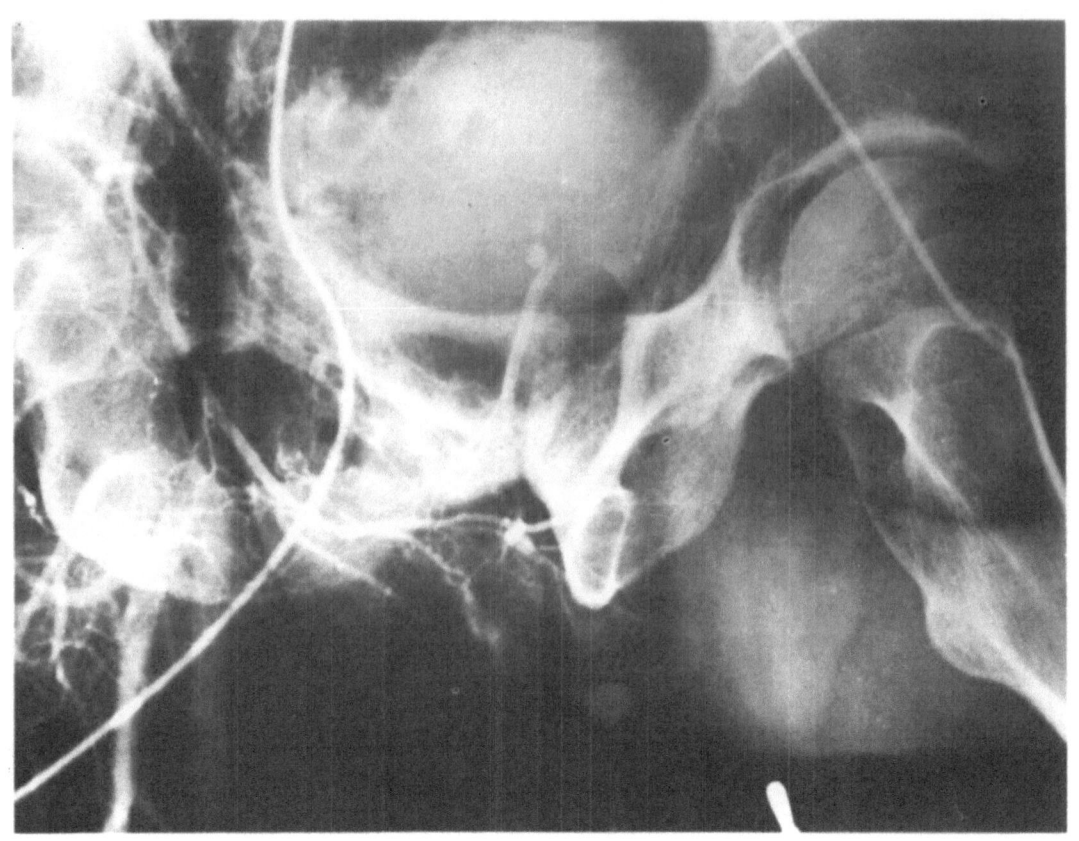

Fig. 51-52 - Amputation of deep artery

No visible pathologic view at level of internal pudendal artery.

Normal aspect of posterior third of deep artery.

Brutal amputation of this artery at union third posterior - third medium.

Posterior cavernogram only exists.

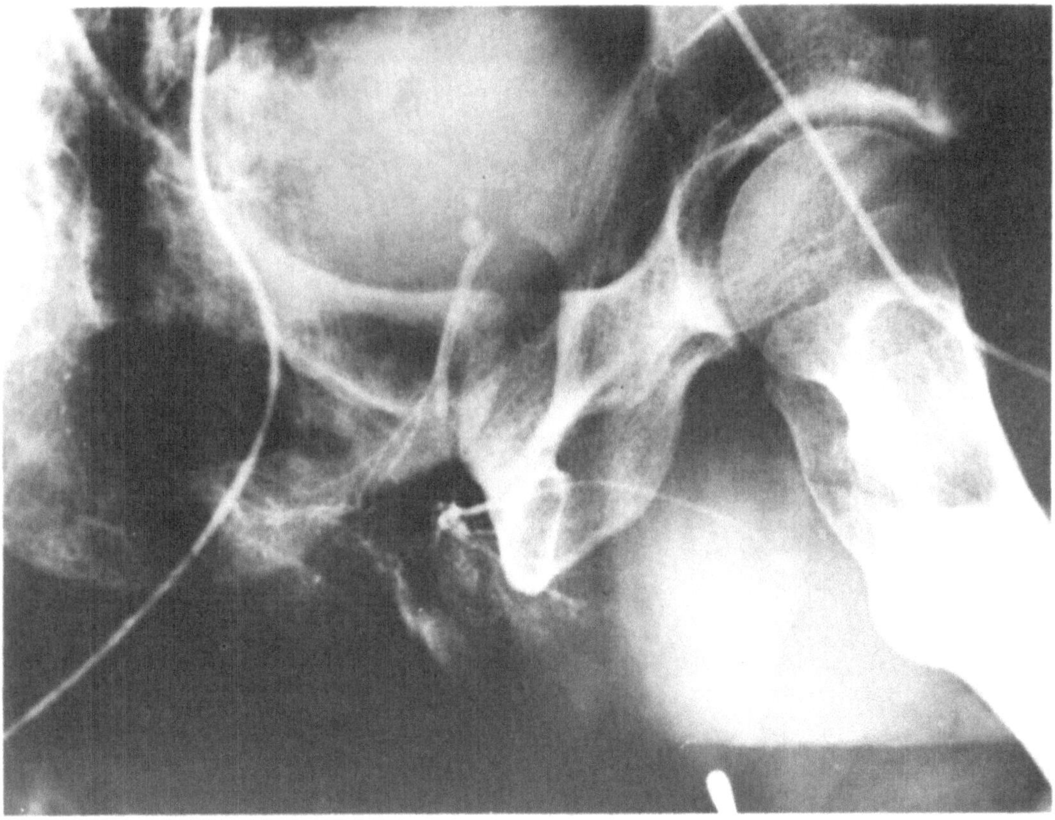

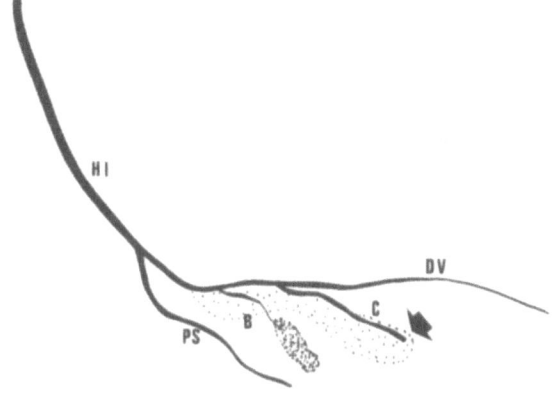

arteriography of internal pudendal artery/**87**

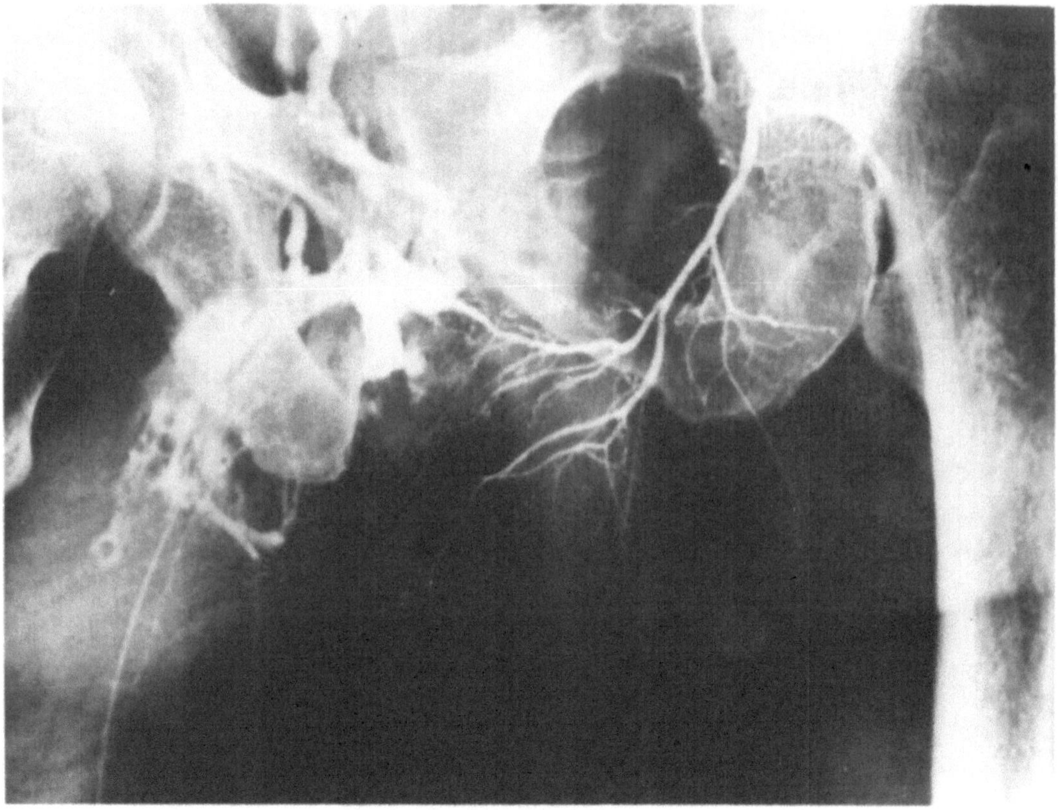

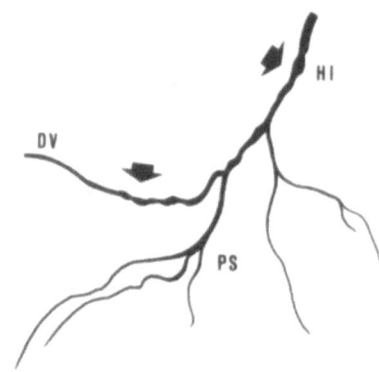

Fig. 53 - Dorsal arteriography of retrograde penis

Atheromatous notches on ischio-rectal segment and perineal segment of internal pudendal artery.

Amputation of artery of penial bulb and deep artery.

III) DISTRIBUTION OF LESIONS ACCORDING TO THE DEGREE OF IMPOTENCE

In order to avoid any misunderstanding with our patients, we have adopted an erection scale going from 0 to 10. Some of the gradations are as follows.

10/10 : normal erection

0/10 : absence of erection

5/10 : lower limit of erection which allows intercourse.

In impotence graded between 0/10 and 3/10 the vascular lesions are always bilateral : bilateral amputation or unilateral amputation with pronounced stenoses on the opposite side.

In impotence graded between 4/10 and 7/10 we may find any of the following :

— unilateral amputation with unaffected opposite axis. Important point : with only one pudendal axis there can be no normal erection ;

— bilateral atheromatous stenoses without amputation ;

— bilateral amputation with distal revascularization ;

— unilateral revascularized amputation and contralateral stenosés in stages ;

— dysplasia.

IV) DISTRIBUTION OF LESIONS ACCORDING TO AGE

In young men without any systemic arterial disease the vascular lesions are always distal ; they are located almost exclusively in the perineal area. An infectious factor is often found.

In older men, apart from lesions of the internal iliac artery, which belong to the iliac group of arteriopathies, the lesions are more diffused, involving most frequently the ischiorectal and perineal portions of the internal pudendal artery and the penile arteries. However, most of the lesions are found in the perineal portion of the internal pudendal artery and the deep artery of the penis.

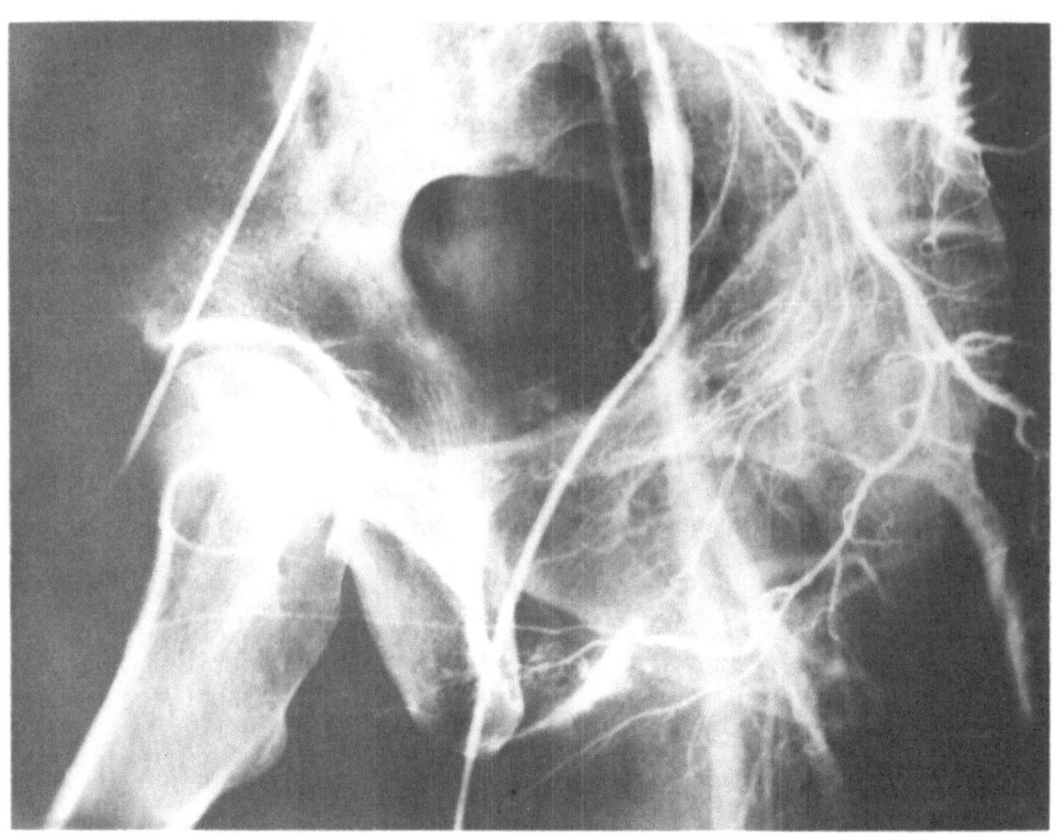

Fig. 54-55 -. Amputation + repermeabilization of deep artery

Amputation of deep artery at third medium level.

Reinjection of distal third by intra-cavernous repermeabilization tracks.

This eventuality is exceptional.

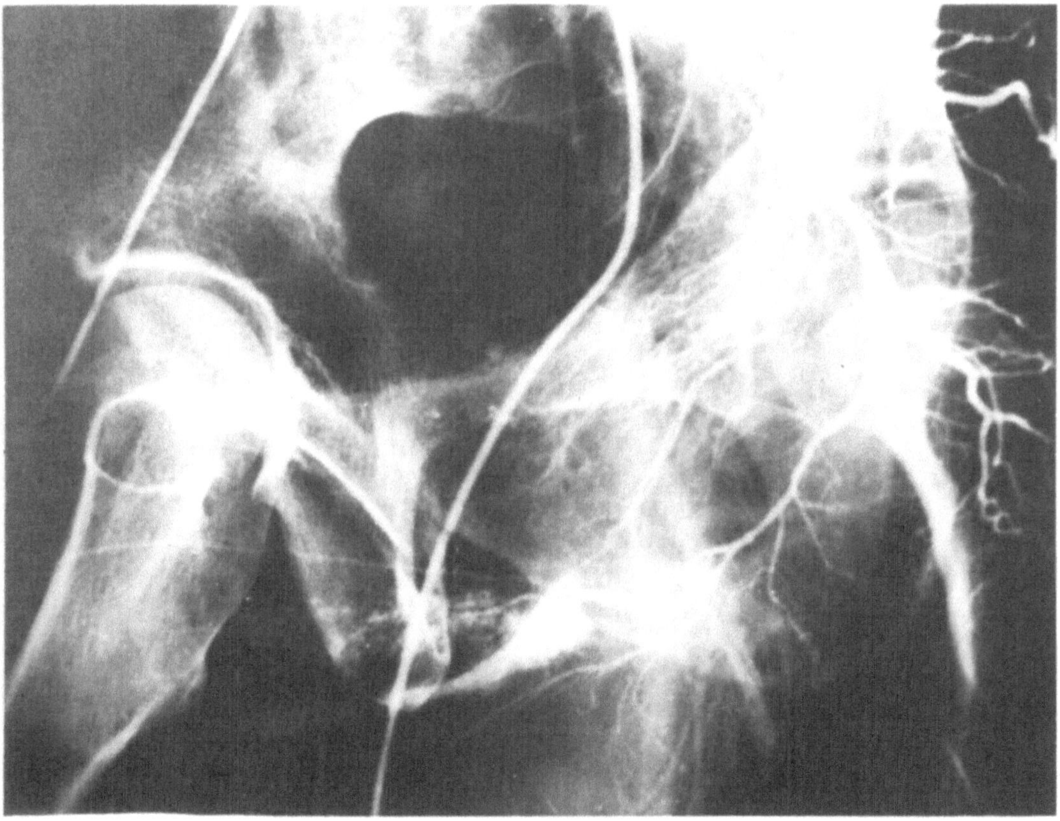

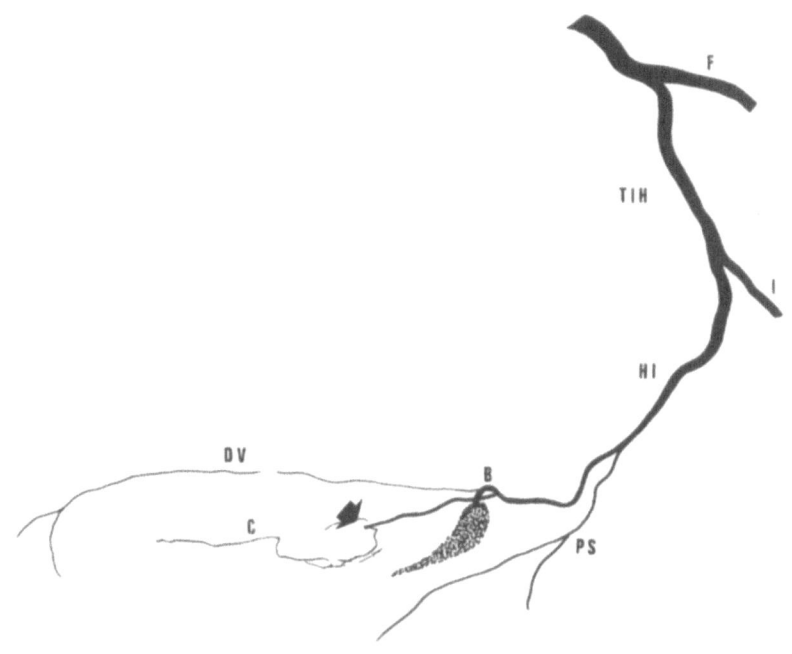

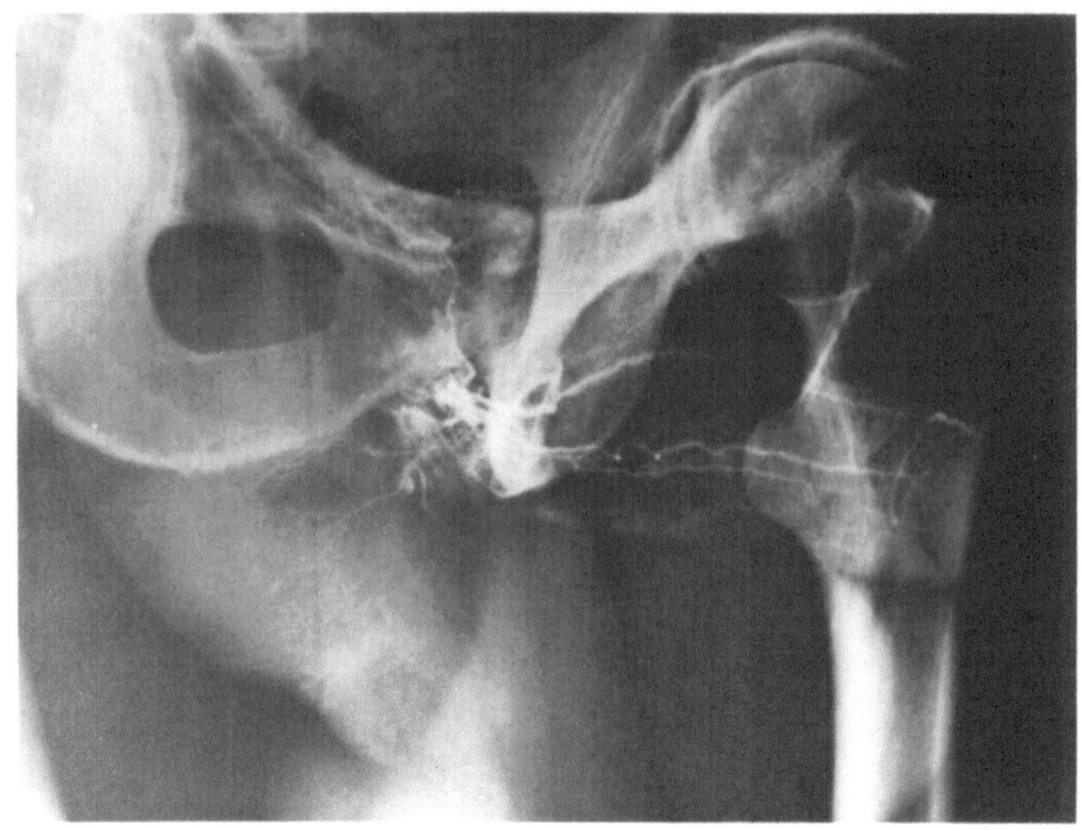

Fig. 56-57 - Dorsal arteriography of retrograde penis

Normal aspect of dorsal artery of penis and deep artery.

Reflux of contrasting fluid in retro-symphysial artery.

No opacification of perineal portion because of its amputation which was the reason motivating this examination.

After a delay of time, very good impregnation of corps cavernosum and corps spongisum.

92/*radiologic exploration of impotence*

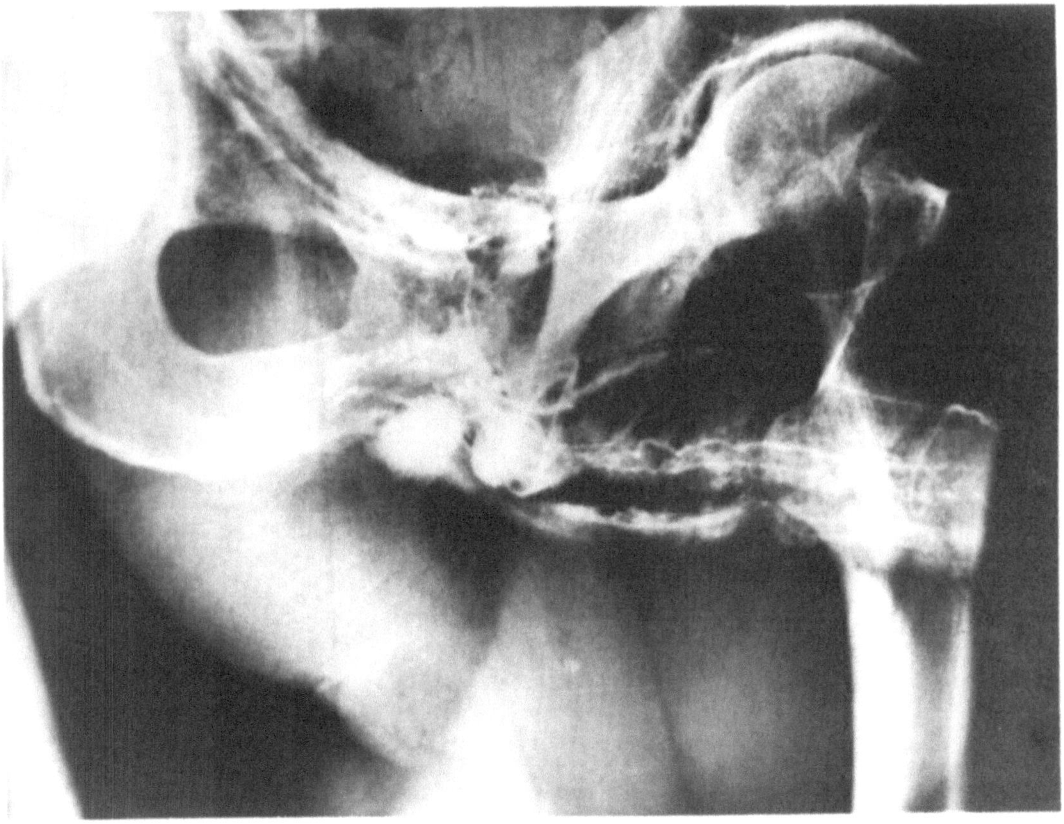

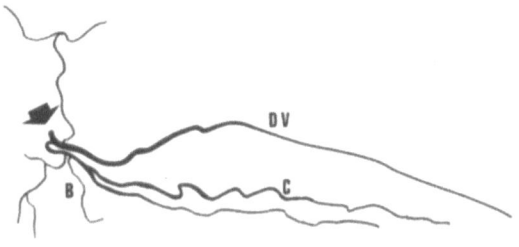

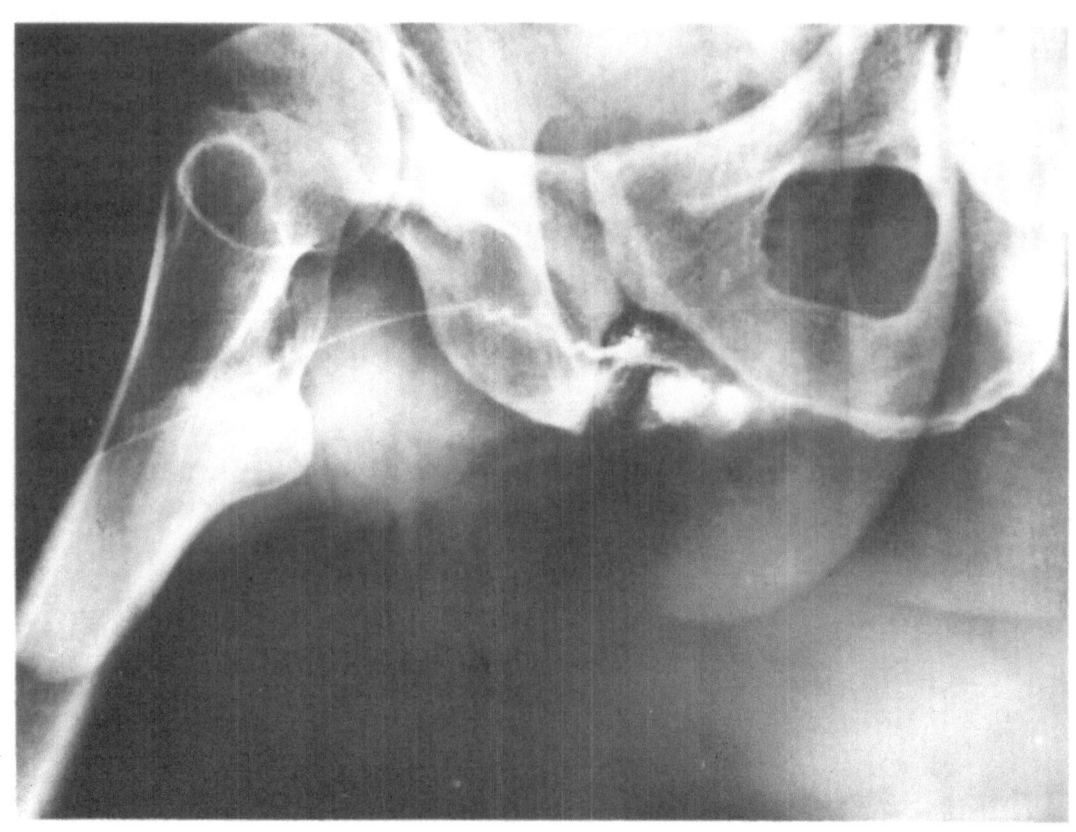

Fig. 58-59 - Dorsal arteriography of retrograde penis
Amputation of deep artery just after its origin.
Normal injection of artery of penial bulb.

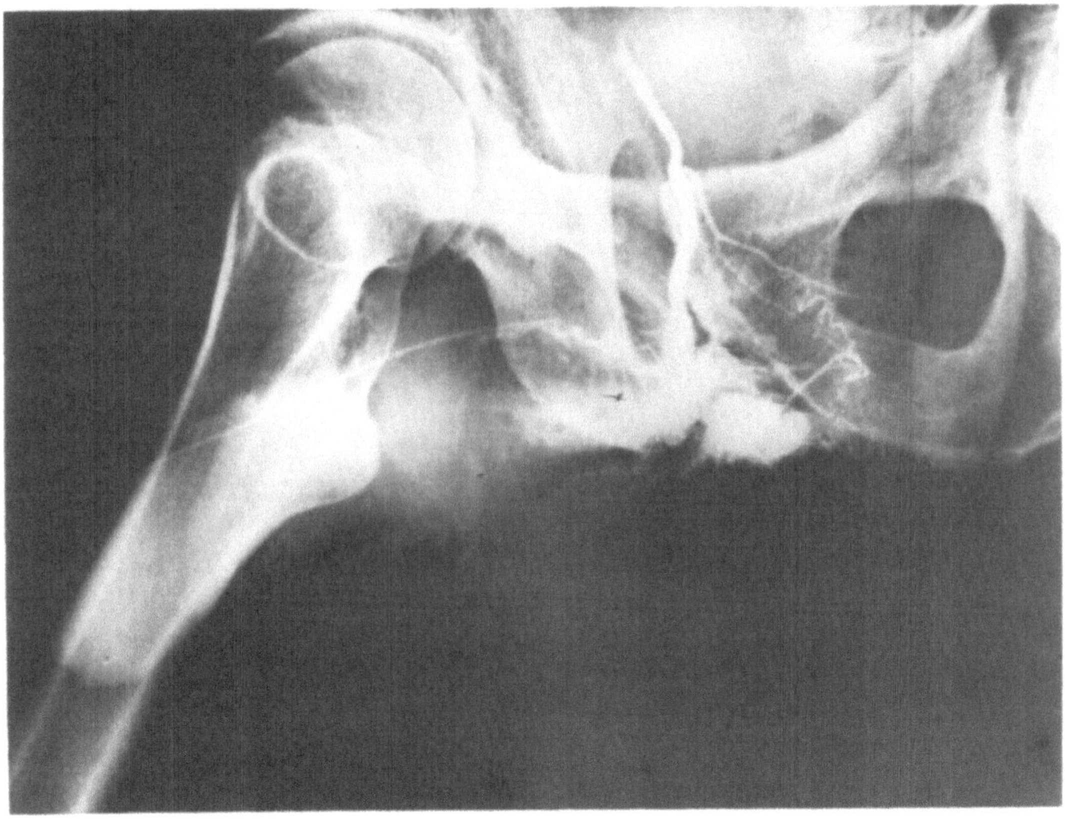

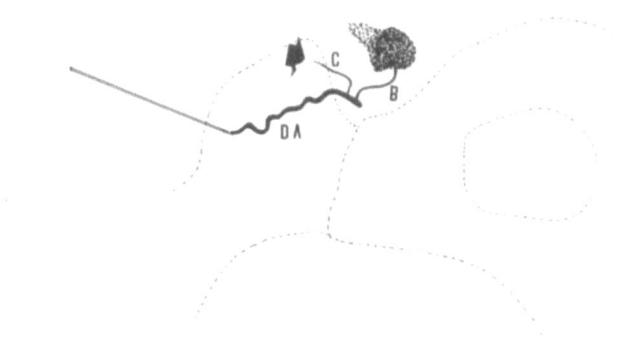

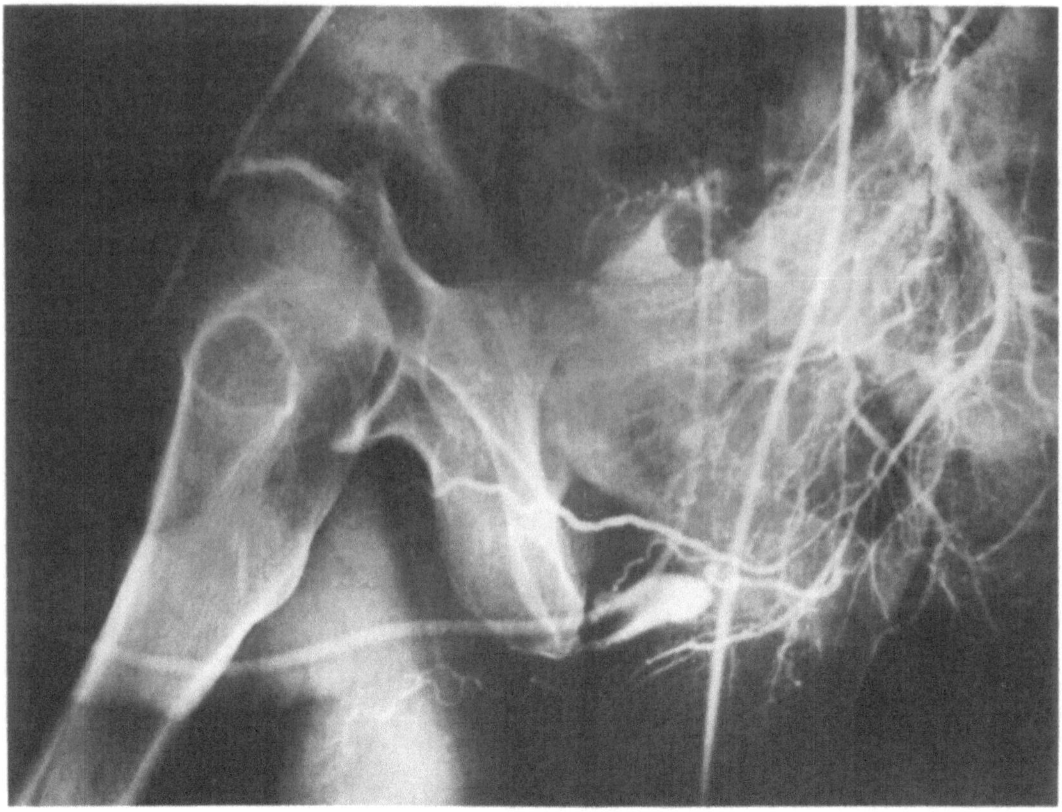

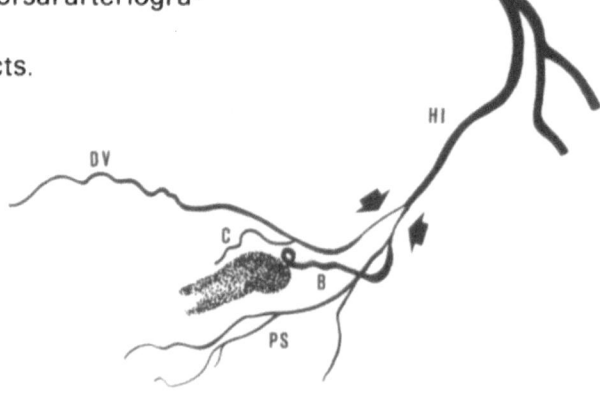

Fig. 60 - Stenoses of internal pudendal artery

Lower part of ischio-rectal segment of internal pudendal artery divides into a dorso-cavernous trunk and a perino-bulbo trunk. The two branches of this inverted Y are equally narrowed. The upstream arteries regain their normal caliber.

Only the origin of the deep artery is opacified.

These views have been verified by dorsal arteriography of the retrograde penis.

It is difficult to classify these aspects.

ETIOLOGY

Three etiologies can be ascertained : atheroma, dysplasia, and infectious thromboangiitis.

Atheroma

In this case, signs are always multiple and analogous to those observed in other arteries of the body : notches and hardening of arterial walls associated or not with pictures of occlusion.

Dysplasia

The widespread aspect of hypotrophy or the absence of injection of certain arterial segments in patients who, since puberty, never had a normal erection cannot easily be related to any acquired lesion.

Infectious thromboangiitis

This is the etiology we should keep in mind in a younger subject with a history of urethritis and prostatitis, when there is a picture of amputation appearing on arteries without any other lesion, in an area where the internal pudendal artery is of small caliber and in contact with the urethral bulb and the prostate.

Other etiologies

A precise etiology cannot be determined for some vascular amputations since it is practically impossible to expose these patients to an arterial biopsy and anatomopathologic studies.

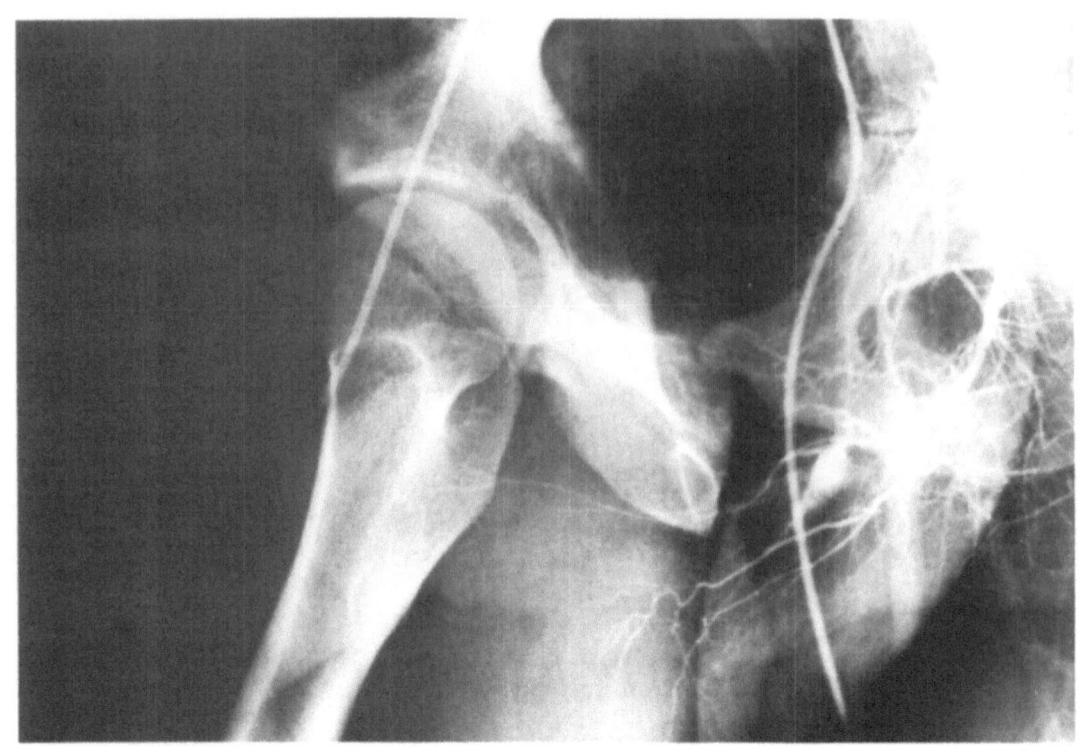

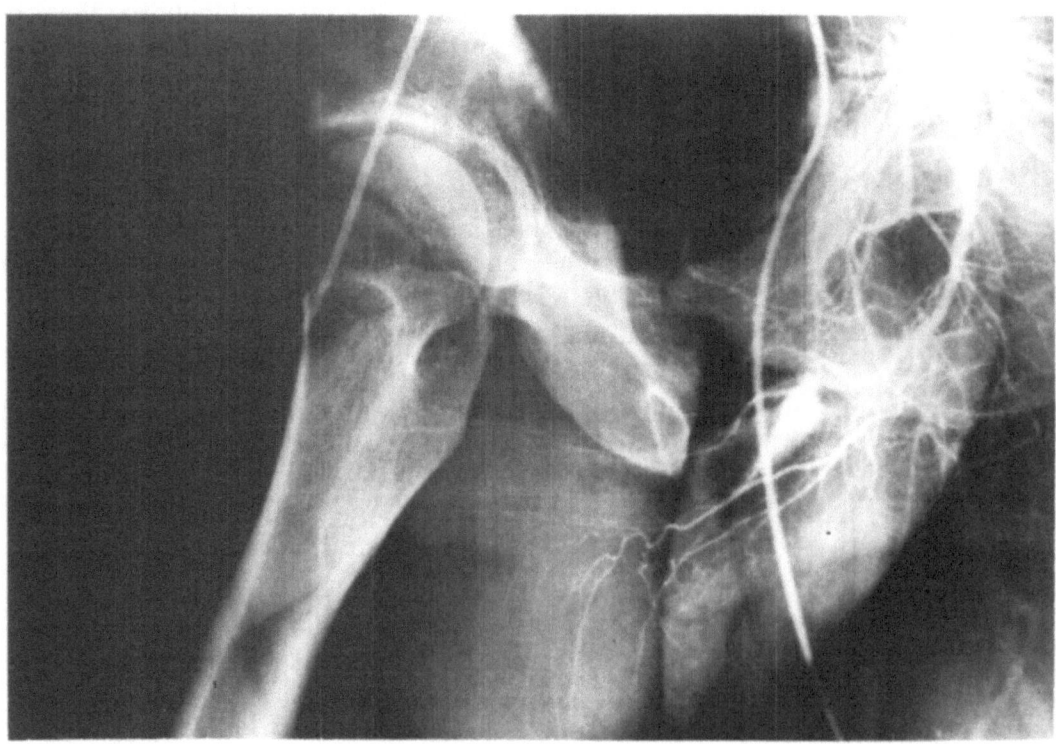

98/*radiologic exploration of impotence*

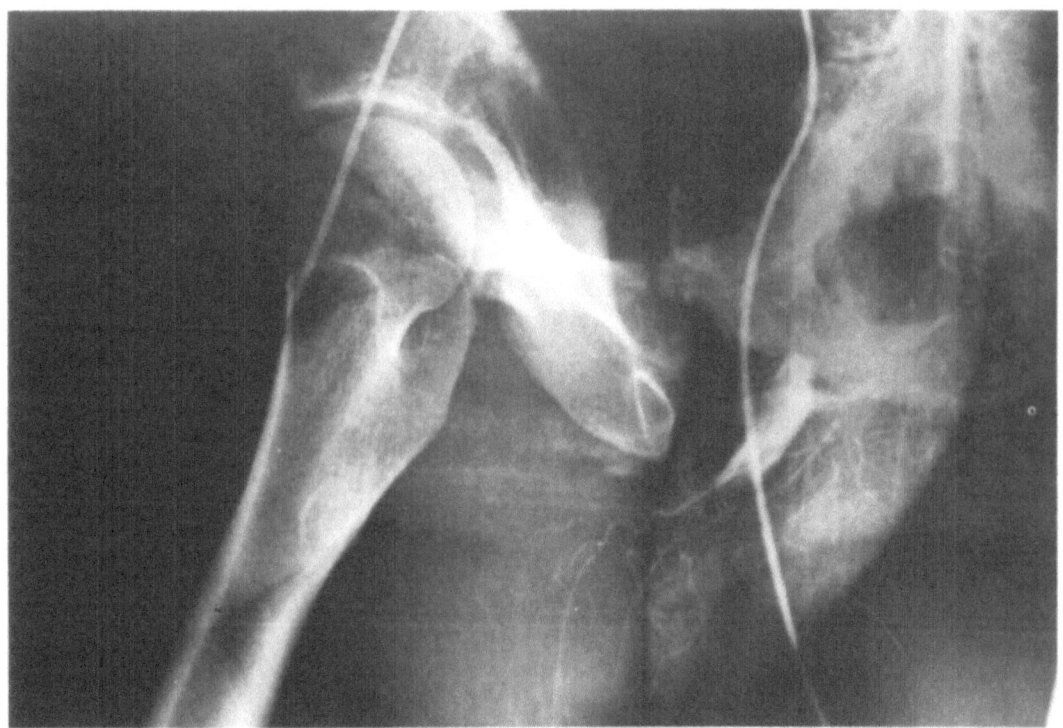

Fig. 61-62-63 - Dysplasia

Patient 20 years old. Has always had soft erection with deviation in penis.

- Arteriography of left internal pudendal :
  - — normal aspect of left internal pudendal artery,
  - — very thin, wirelike aspect of deep artery, totally visible.

Dorsal artery of penis, which is as thin as deep artery and is only visible at its proximal half level.

- Arteriography of right internal pudendal :
  - — no pathologic view,
  - — no compensatory hypertrophy.

- Dorsal arteriography of left retrograde penis
  - — was impossible. When denuded, dorsal artery of penis was of such small caliber that it was not possible to catherize, even with a lymphotography catheter.

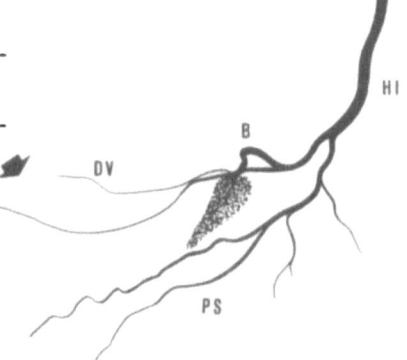

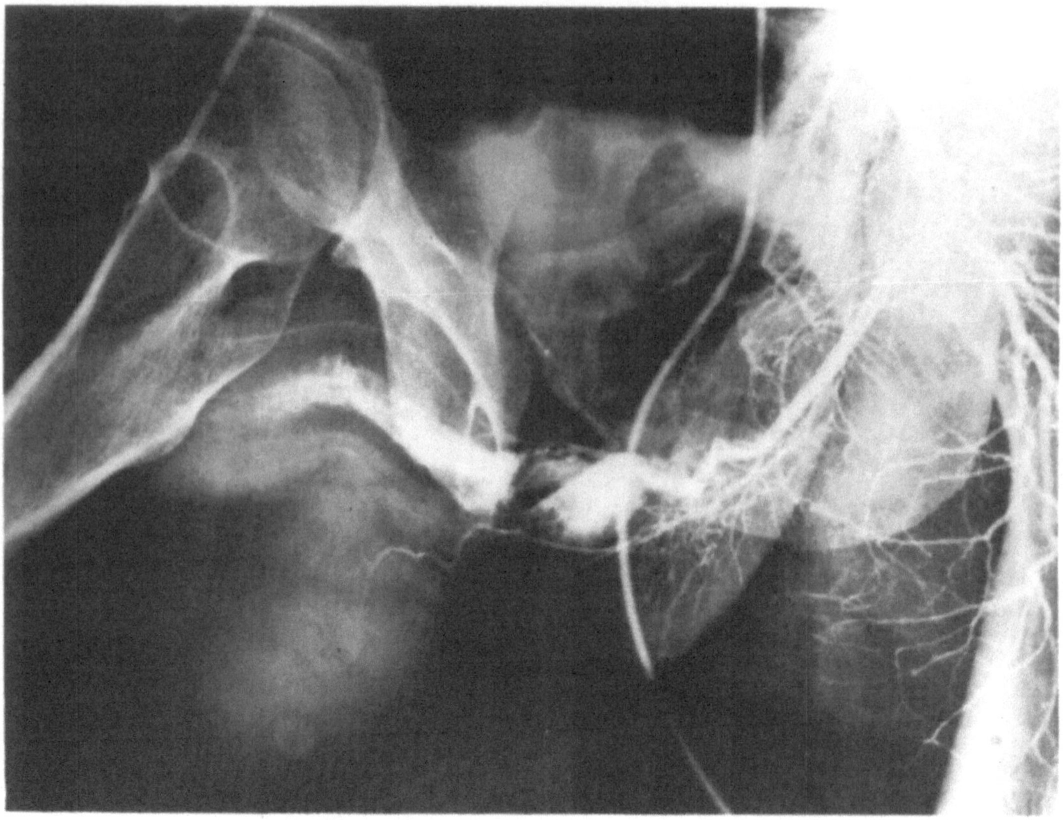

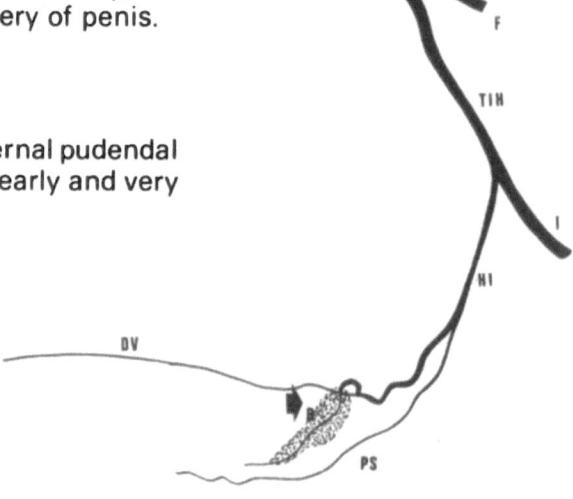

Fig. 64-65-66 - Arterial dysplasia

Left side :

— Normal aspect of internal pudendal artery, artery of panial bulb, and dorsal artery of penis.
— Agenesia of deep artery.

Right side :

— Compensatory hypertrophy of internal pudendal artery, and of deep artery, with very early and very dense cavernogrophy.

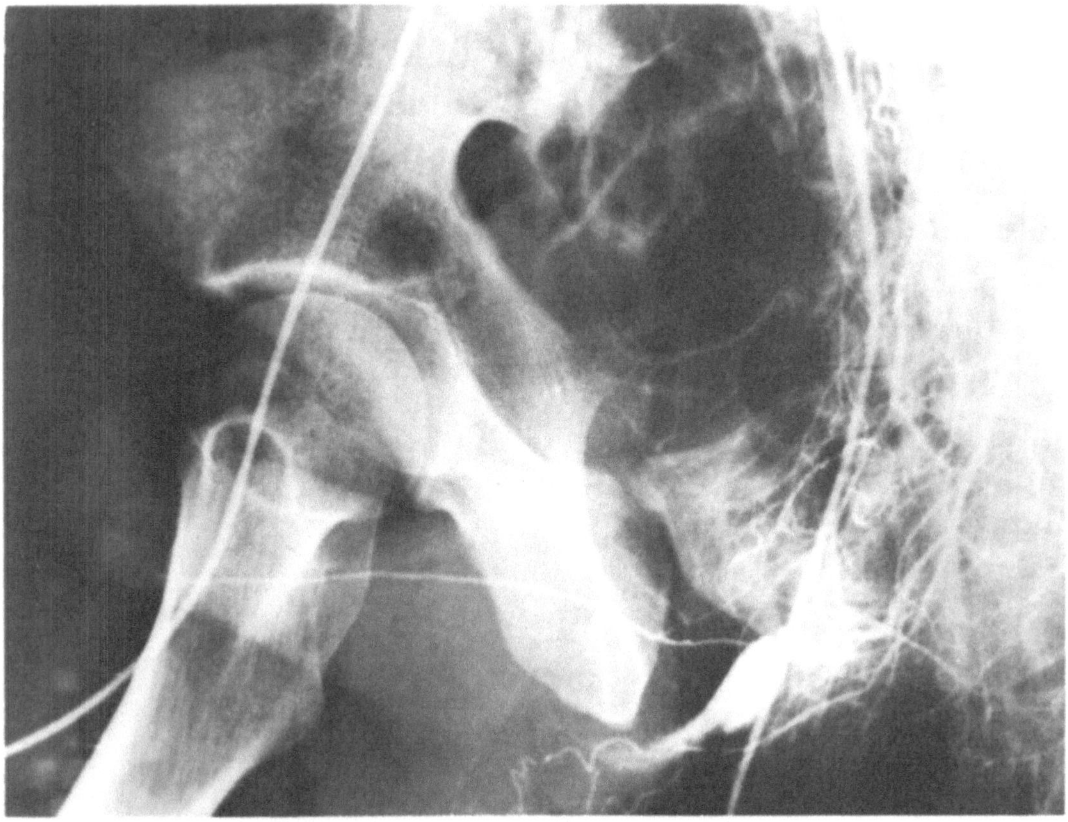

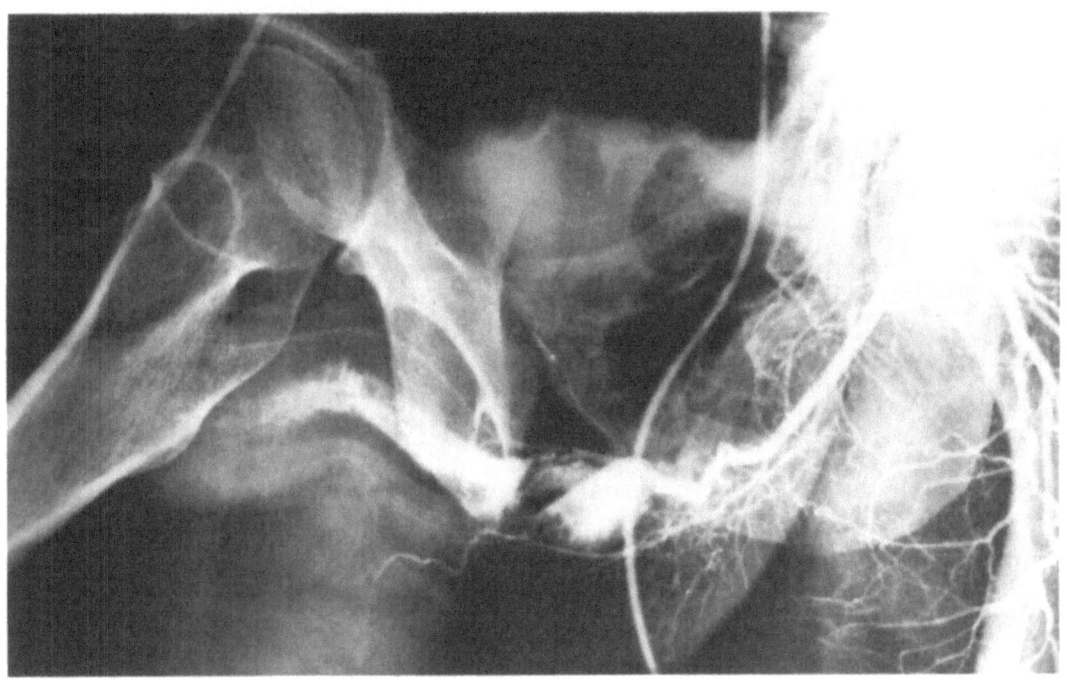

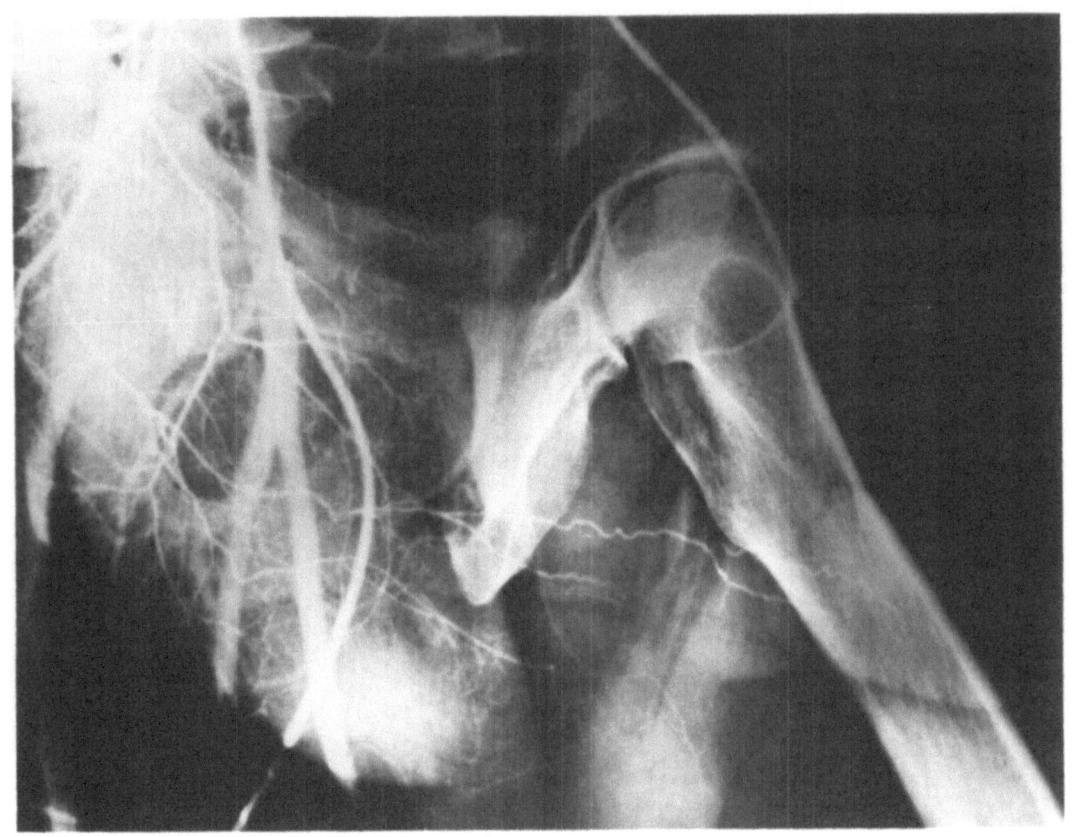

Fig. 67-68 - Thin aspect of internal pudendal artery

Thin aspect but regular aspect of internal pudendal artery and its branches.

Absence of precise hemodynamics tests make it difficult to appreciate the value of such views.

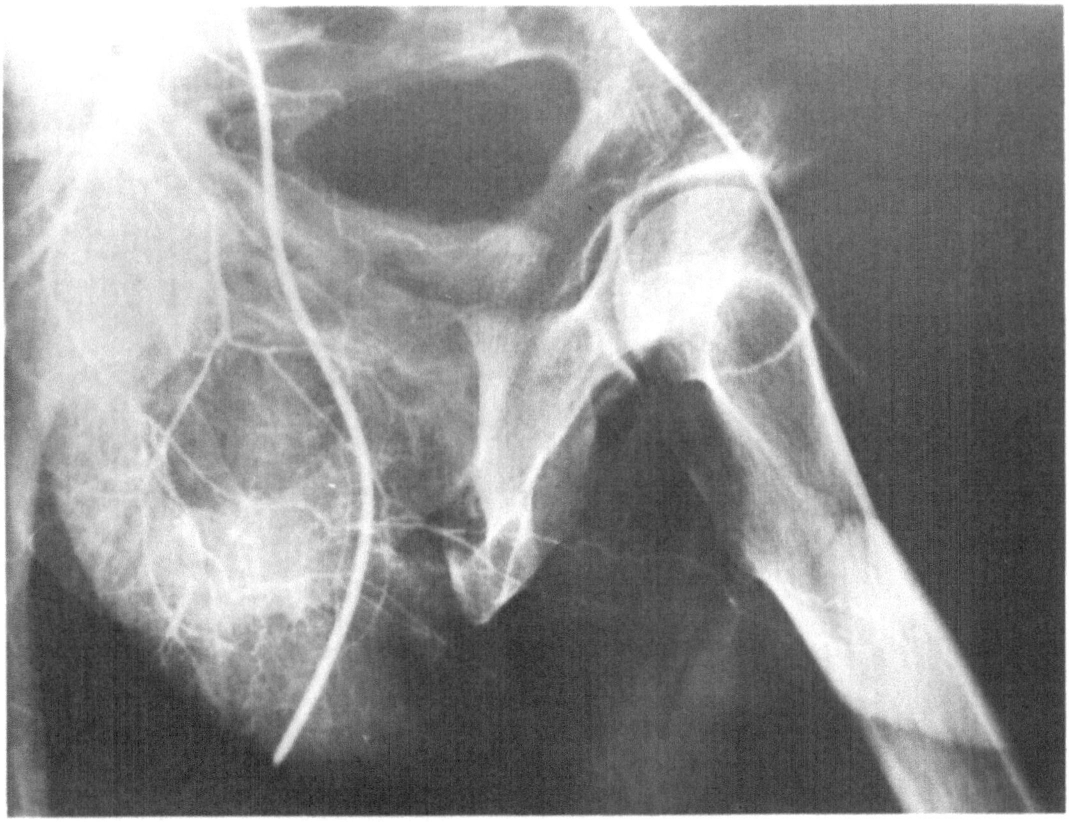

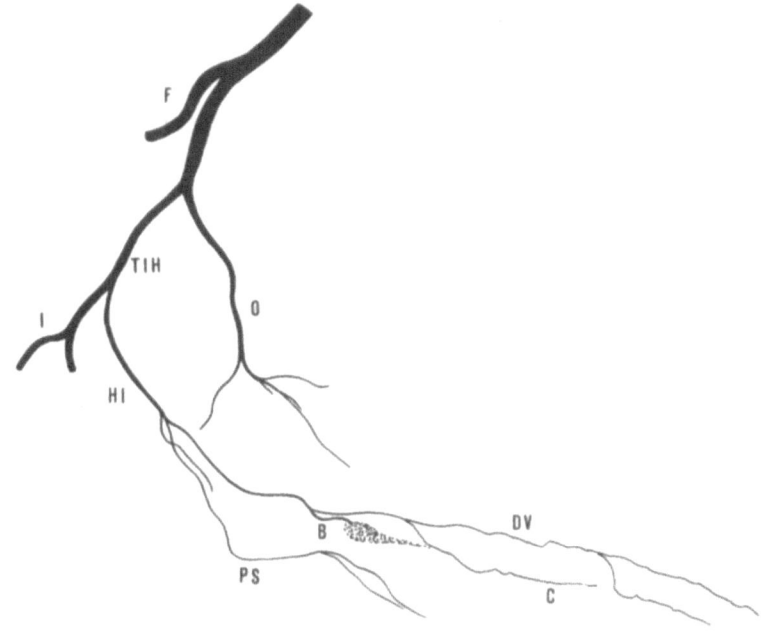

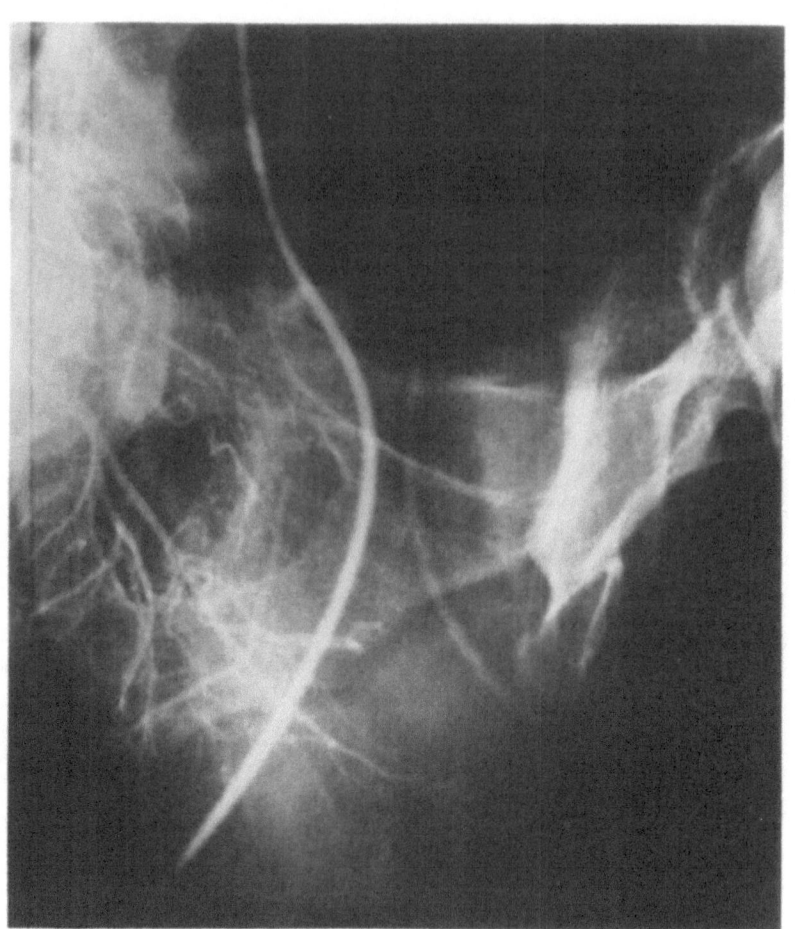

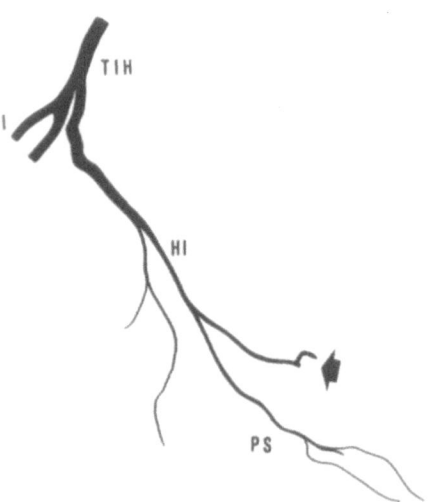

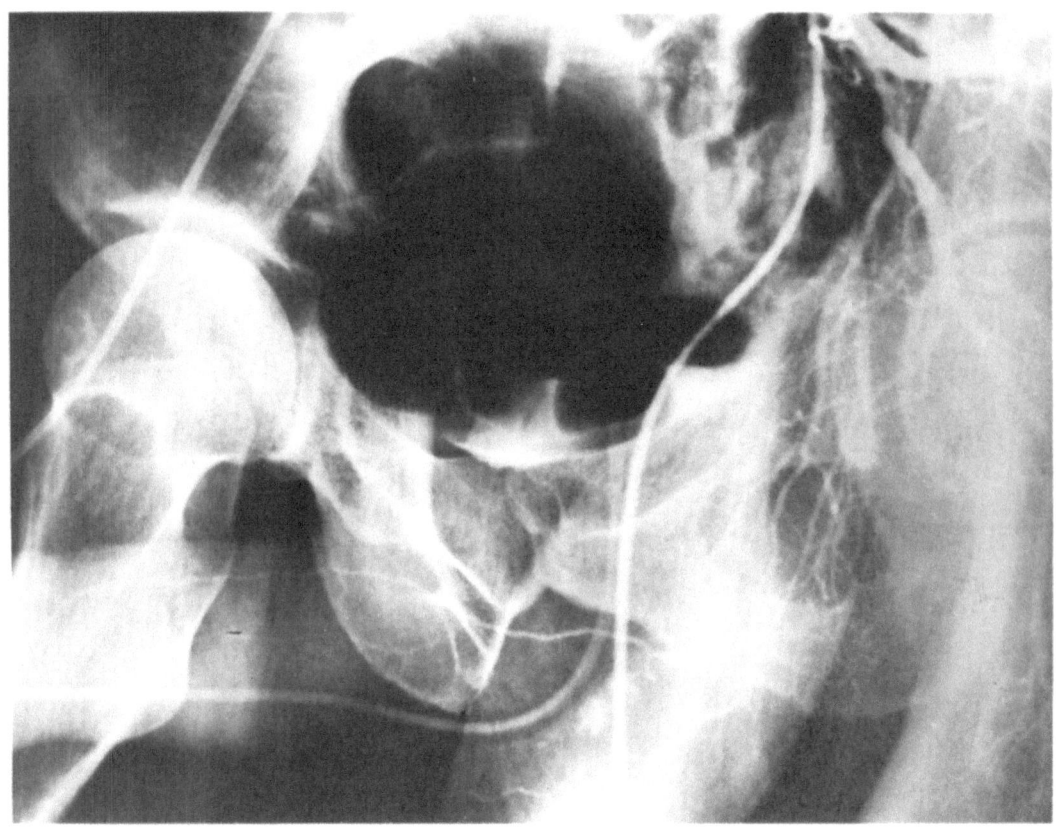

Fig. 69-70 - Amputation of internal pudental artery

Patient 40 year old man. Brutal onset of impotence (4/10) after a brucellien prostatsis.

Right internal pudendal artery : amputation of artery at origin of its perineal portion.

Normal aspect of left internal pudendal artery.

Hyphothesis of obliteration thrombo-angeitis at contact of an infectious foyer should be considered.

ARTERIOGRAPHY OF INTERNAL PUDENDAL ARTERY

INDICATIONS

I) **INDICATIVE CLINICAL PICTURE**

II) **ETIOLOGIES TO BE RULED OUT**

III) **THERAPEUTIC PERSPECTIVES**

At present, pelvic and abdominal arteriographies are practically without any complications, provided they be done by a cautious and competent operator. However, they remain serious radiologic explorations and their indications must be carefully studied. That is why the following conditions must be fulfilled.

1) The clinical picture is indicative of an arterial etiology
2) Other etiologies have been ruled out
3) The therapeutic outlook is good.

I) INDICATIVE CLINICAL PICTURE

The clinical picture is quite revealing. In complete absence of erection none occurs in spite of the patient's desire of sexual intercourse and none during the night or in the morning.

In insufficient erection the patients have soft erections in their attempts at intercourse, and no erection or soft erections during the night or upon awakening.

Sometimes there is a variation in the clinical picture. Some of these patients achieve inconsistently, when recumbent, a nearly normal erection which vanishes upon a change of position. This is due to the increase of blood flow in the superior and inferior gluteal and the external iliac arteries occuring upon change of position at the expense of the arteries supplying the pelvis. This hemodynamic change decompensates the territories of the pudendal pathways.

Impotence is a clinical sign. As such it requires a complete examination of the patient as well as complementary laboratory investigations in order to reveal or eliminate certain etiologies of impotence which we shall not discuss in this monograph. We mention only briefly the following.

Neurologic Etiology

Beside the well-known syndromes of spinal cord injury and of the cauda equina there are other etiologies, the diagnoses of which are currently being studied by several medical teams in France.

Impotence secondary to amputation of the rectum has conventionally been considered as of neurologic origin. It is however possible that there is in certain cases a vascular cause or component whose origin is also surgical. We did not have the opportunity to examine such patients by arteriography ; those referred to us refused to submit to this exploration.

Medicamentous etiology

Three main groups of drugs are responsible : psychotropics, antihypertensives, and L-dopa.

● *Psychotropic drugs*

Most patients who had previously psychiatric treatment take psychotropic drugs in smaller or larger doses. Before it is possible to make a thorough clinical and laboratory examination, it is imperative to wean such patients progressively, though completely, away from their drugs. If this is not possible, an exploration is useless.

● *Antihypertensive drugs*

They all can cause impotence. This puts the patient before the dilemma of choosing between the treatment of his arterial hypertension and the chance of recovering a normal sexual activity.

● *L-Dopa and its derivatives*

L-dopa is a stimulant of erection at small doses, but becomes a cause of impotence if taken in larger doses.

Metabolic etiology

The metabolic disorders that should be looked for in particular are hyperuricemia and hyperlipidemia.

Hematologic etiology

All conditions of hyperviscosity of the blood can be causes of impotence. The most typical example is polycythemia. The related impotence regresses with treatment.

Endocrine etiology

Although hormonal causes are the most classical, they are relatively infrequent. In a diabetic patient impotence is considered to be caused by diabetic neuropathy. It would however be useful to make a certain number of arteriograms in such patients in order to find whether there might not be some distal lesion in the internal pudendal or the deep penile artery. Such a lesion would manifest itself much earlier than in the extremities, because at the level of the pudendal arteries there are no such large and numerous physiologic anastomoses as there are at the level of the arteires in the hands and feet.

Renal etiology

Hyperazotemia can cause impotence. In patients who are undergoing renal dialysis the cause does not seem to be psychiatric, as certain authors have written, but vascular or medicamentous. This question is further being studied at present.

Psychiatric etiology

We recognize from the beginning as psychiatric patient every subject who presents a behavioral disorder other than his problem of sexual behavior.

III) THERAPEUTIC PERSPECTIVES

When the clinical picture is clear and the other etiologies of impotence have been ruled out, the indication for arteriography should be established in so far as it can lead to a therapeutic program for the patient.

This therapeutic program, medical or surgical, demands in either case the participation of the patient's partner in order to have the best chances of success. Sexual pathology, as we have pointed out in the Introduction, is a pathology of relationship. The pathologic condition of one person infers a secondary, « reactional » pathologic status in his or her partner.

Therefore, the partner must be examined, and possibly treated, at the same time as the impotent patient, so that the latter does not have to deal, at the threshold of his cure, with the female pathology (frigidity, vaginism) he himself induced.

Resumption of sexual intercourse will not immediately be normal and can never again become completely normal. It is indispensable that the female partner be aware of the male's problem and that she participate in the therapy.

When the indications for arteriography are established according to the above-mentioned principles, the arteriographic findings are positive in 93 per cent of the cases.

CAVERNOGRAPHY

I) **TECHNIQUE**

- — Puncture of the corpora cavernosa
- — Projections
- — Opacification
- — Recording

II) **NORMAL RŒNTGEN ANATOMY**

III) **PATHOLOGIC RŒNTGEN ANATOMY**

TECHNIQUE

I) PUNCTURE OF THE CORPORA CAVERNOSA

The puncture of only one corpus cavernosum is necessary, thanks to large and numerous communications between the two cavernous bodies. For this puncture we use a simple 18 G scalp vein catheter.

After disinfection of the skin of the penis, the cavernous body is punctured on its dorsal aspect, at the level of its distal third. The puncture must be done quite obliquely so as to avoid to traverse the entire width of the cavernous body and to enter the corpus spongiosum or the urethra. The puncture of the albuginea gives a very definite sensation of venous resistance.

The catheterization of a corpus cavernosum is normally accompanied by a reflux of blood into the catheter. Sometimes it is necessary to provoke this reflux by the injection of a few milliliters of physiologic solution into the catheter after having entered the cavernous body.

II) PROJECTIONS

The basic projection is the ascending oblique, the penis being reclined on the abdomen, as described in the chapter of complementary projections in internal pudendal arteriography. This projection allows a clear differentiation between the left and the right cavernous bodies. It is the only projection that outlines the cavernous bodies from their perineal insertions to their penile extremities.

A lateral projection may be added in order tot demonstrate abnormal curvatures of the penis.

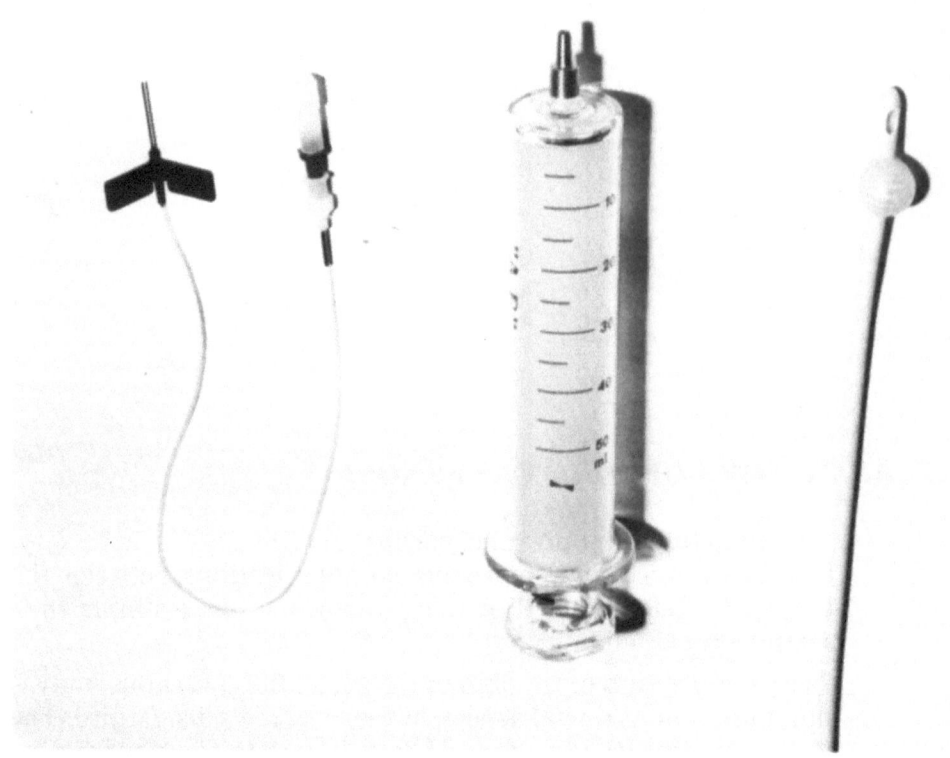

Fig. 71 - Material used for cavernogrophy
Vesicular catheter with ballon.

« Butterfly » scalp vein catheter for corps cavernosum puncture.

Seringue for manual injection.

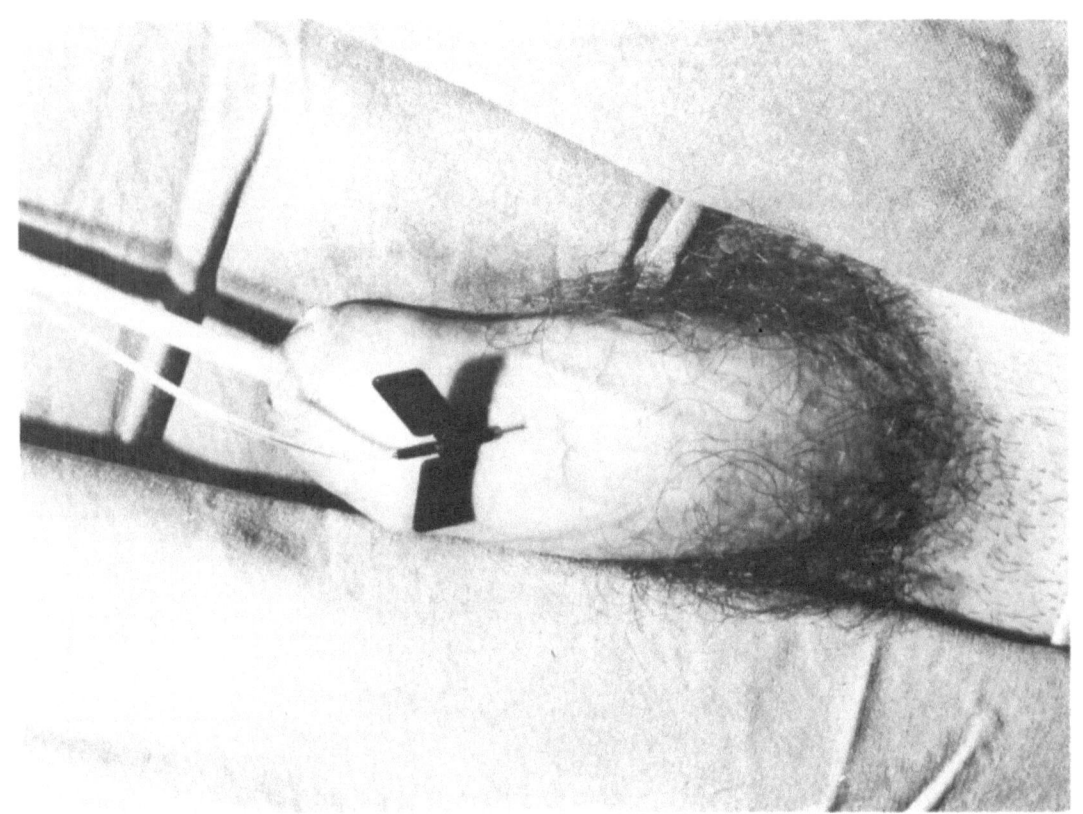

Fig. 72 - Cavernography - puncture

Patient is catheterized.

After skin disinfection, a corps cavernosum is punctured, at its distal portion.

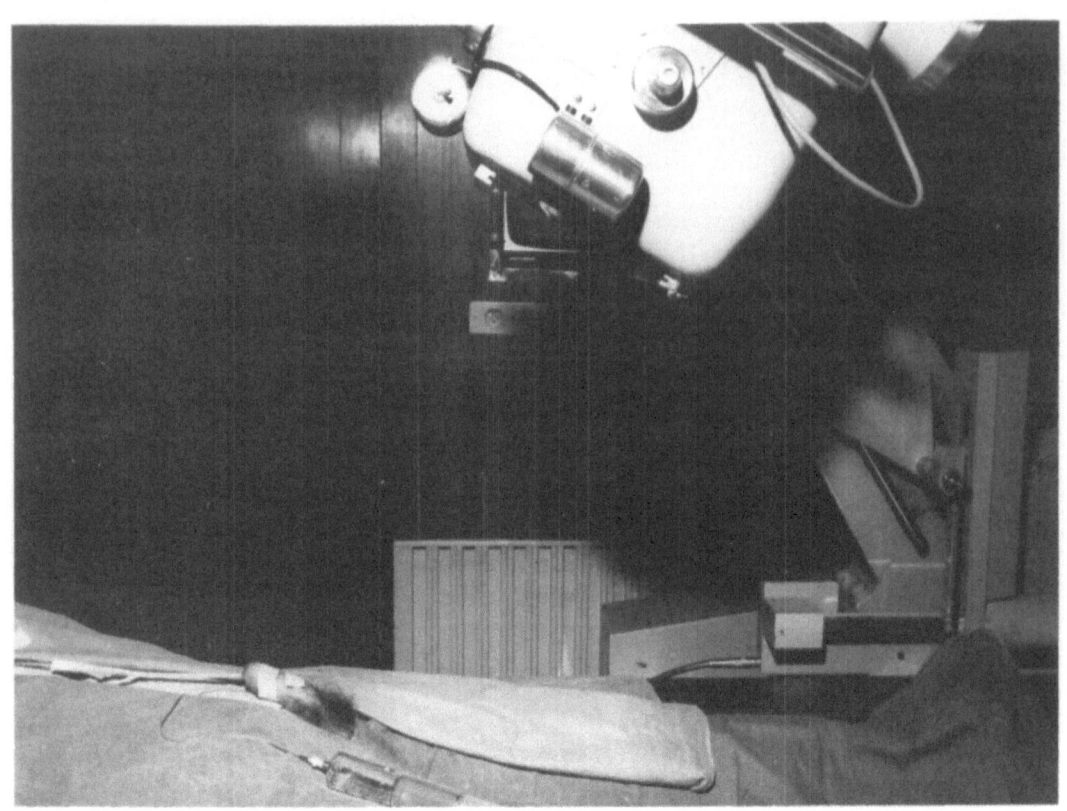

Fig. 73 - Cavernography - position

Penis reclines on abdomen.

X ray beam placed in ascending oblique position.

III) OPACIFICATION

The contrast fluid must be a hydrosoluble substance of relatively low viscosity. We use preheated Télébrix 30 and inject slowly, at the rate of 4 milliliters per second, a total of 40 milliliters.

IV) RECORDING

A 35-cm serialograph is needed. Films are taken at the rate of 1 per second during 15 seconds, the start of the exposures coinciding with the beginning of the injection. The first films allow to study the filling of the corpora cavernosa and the anastomoses between the two corpora. The intermediate films allow a morphologic study of the corpora cavernosa. The late films are to study the venous drainage of the corpora.

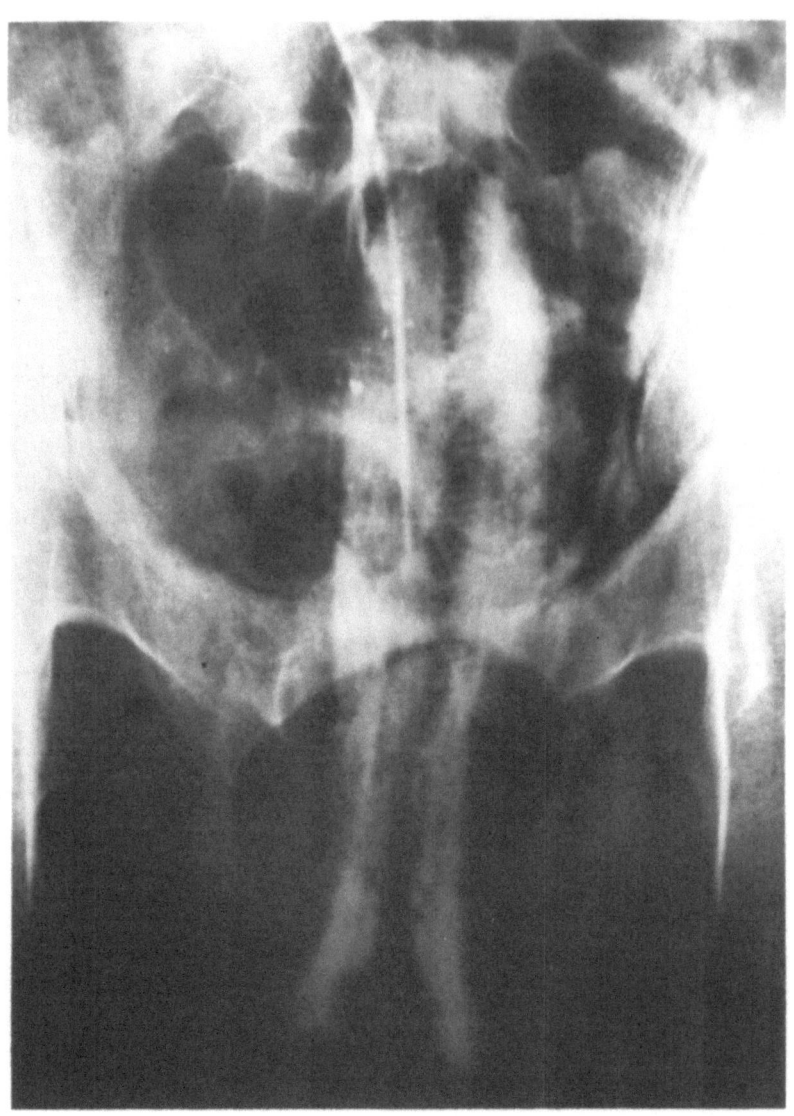

Fig. 74 - Normal cavernography

These views made during opacification show total and symetric vision of two corps cavernosum and numerous vascular anastomoses which connect the two corps cavernosum across the penis septum.

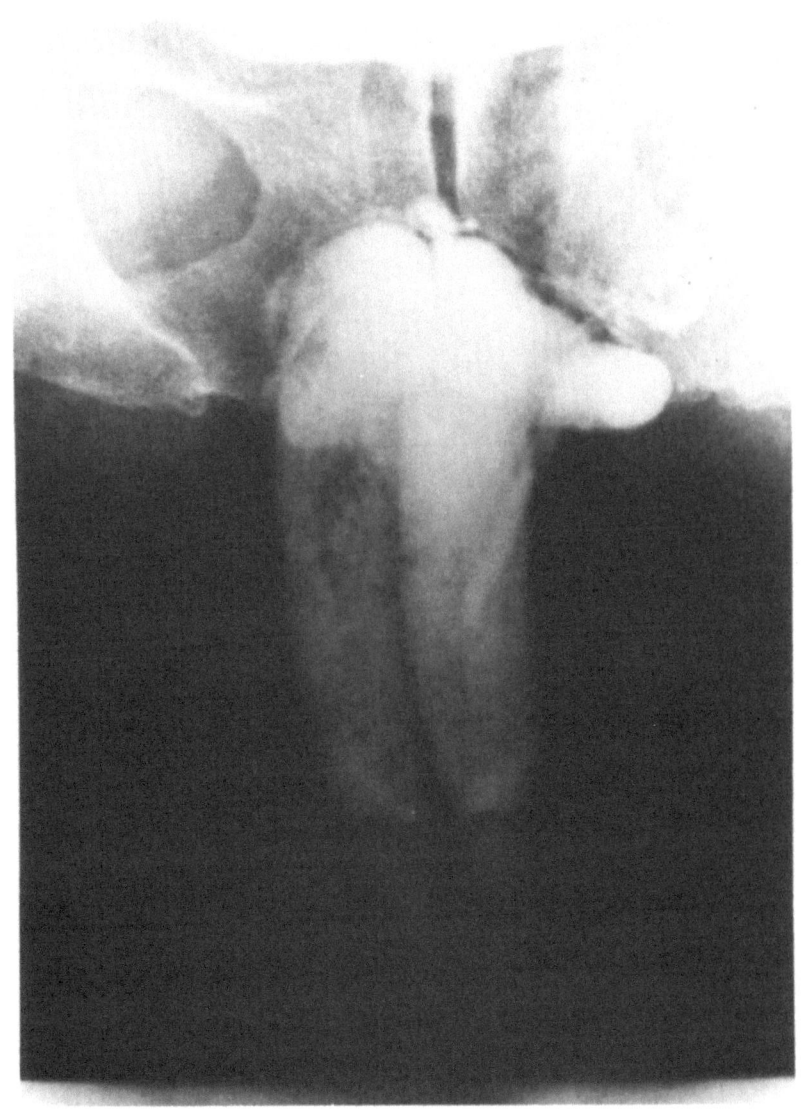

Fig. 75 - Normal cavernography

Symetric injection of two corps cavernosum in spite of unilateral punction.

It concerns late views (5 mn) which show the stagnation of the contrasting fluid in the corps cavernosum.

NORMAL RŒNTGEN ANATOMY

There are two corpora cavernosa which are to be studied from the ischiopubic rami to the posterior aspect of the glans. They are separated from each other by the septum penis which is traversed by numerous and large anastomoses. They are straight, with parallel borders ; the lateral border may be slightly convex. The posterior part of each corpus has the shape of a racket and is oblique posterolaterally. Its anterior extremity is harmoniously convex. The two corpora are symmetric in length and diameter.

The delay in the opacification of the nonpunctured corpus cavernosum as compared to the punctured one is small. At the time of complete filling their opacity is homogeneous.

The venous drainage takes place essentially through the deep dorsal vein of the penis toward Santorini's plexus and the internal iliac (hypogastric) veins.

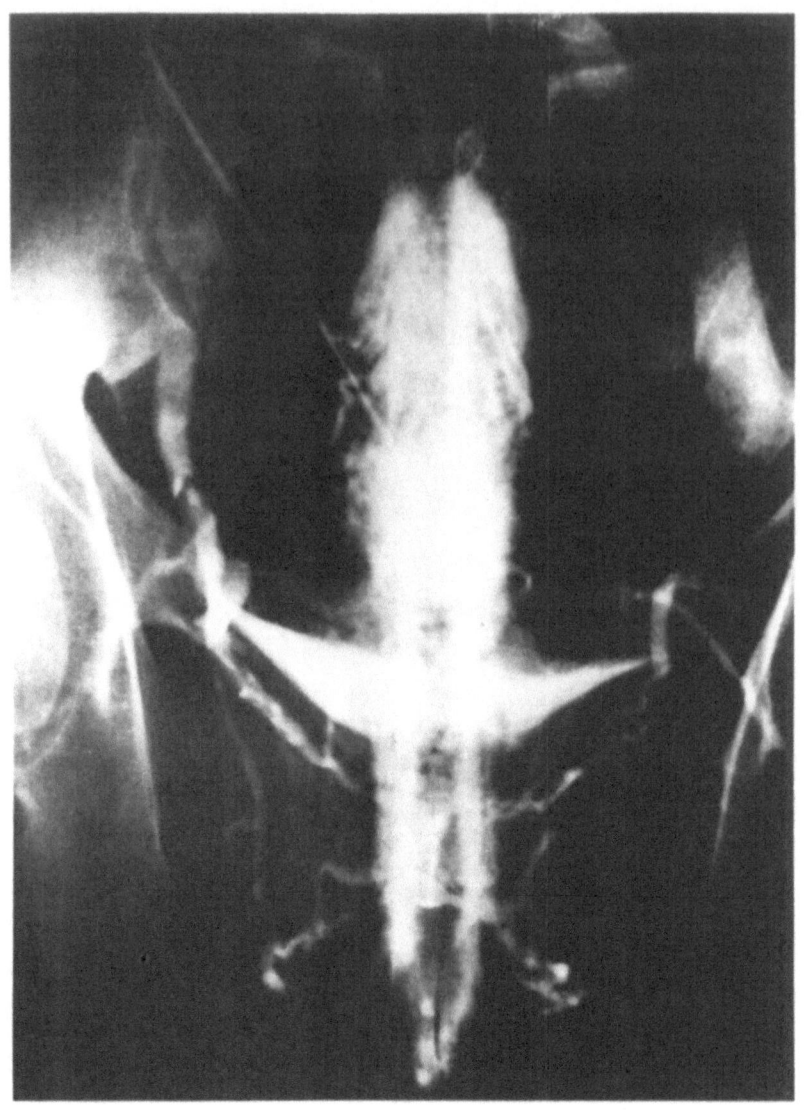

Fig. 76 - Phlebography of corps spongiosum

Realized by punction, on ventral side of penis, of corps spongiosum.

Allows opacification of corps spongiosum and of gland.

It is not further developped in this work for it does not bring any diagnostic teaching.

PATHOLOGIC RŒNTGEN ANATOMY

So far we have observed pathologic changes only in Peyronie's disease, priapism being excluded from this study. The pathologic images are of four types :

— Notches at the level of the albuginea, indicative of a fibrotic lesion :

— Lacunar images at the level of the corpora cavernosa.

— Lack of expansion of part or the total of one or both of the corpora cavernosa.

— Delay in the spreading of the contrast fluid in the corpora cavernosa.

We believe that there is great value in cavernography for the assessment of Peyronie's disease, because it demonstrates the lesions involving both the albuginea and the cavernous bodies. It helps to determine the exact moment at which to operate and to suggest to the patient a treatment before the fibrotic process of the albuginea and the corpora cavernosa be too much advanced to preserve an acceptable degree of erection.

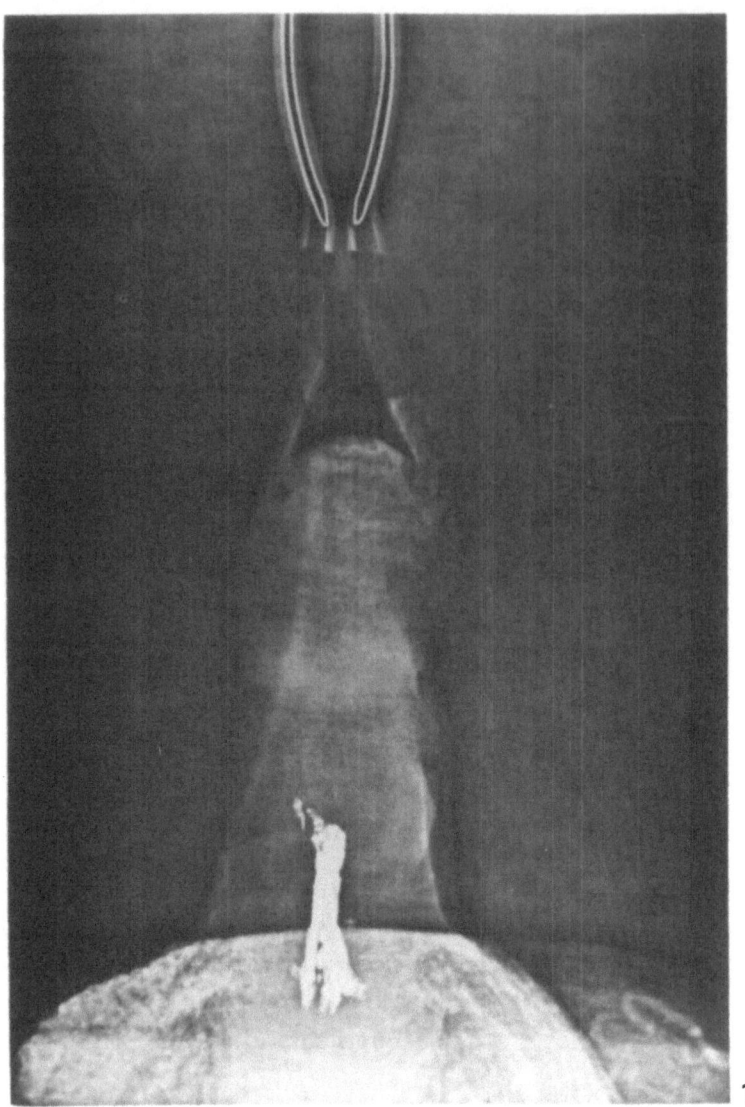

Fig. 77-78 - Peyronie's disease

1) *Xeroradiography :* voluminous perineal calcification.

2) *Cavernography :* multi-lacunal aspect of witness corps cavernosum of intra-cavernous fibroses. Very important transversal lacunal view on penial portion of corps cavernosum on left side, secondary to albuginea fibrosis.

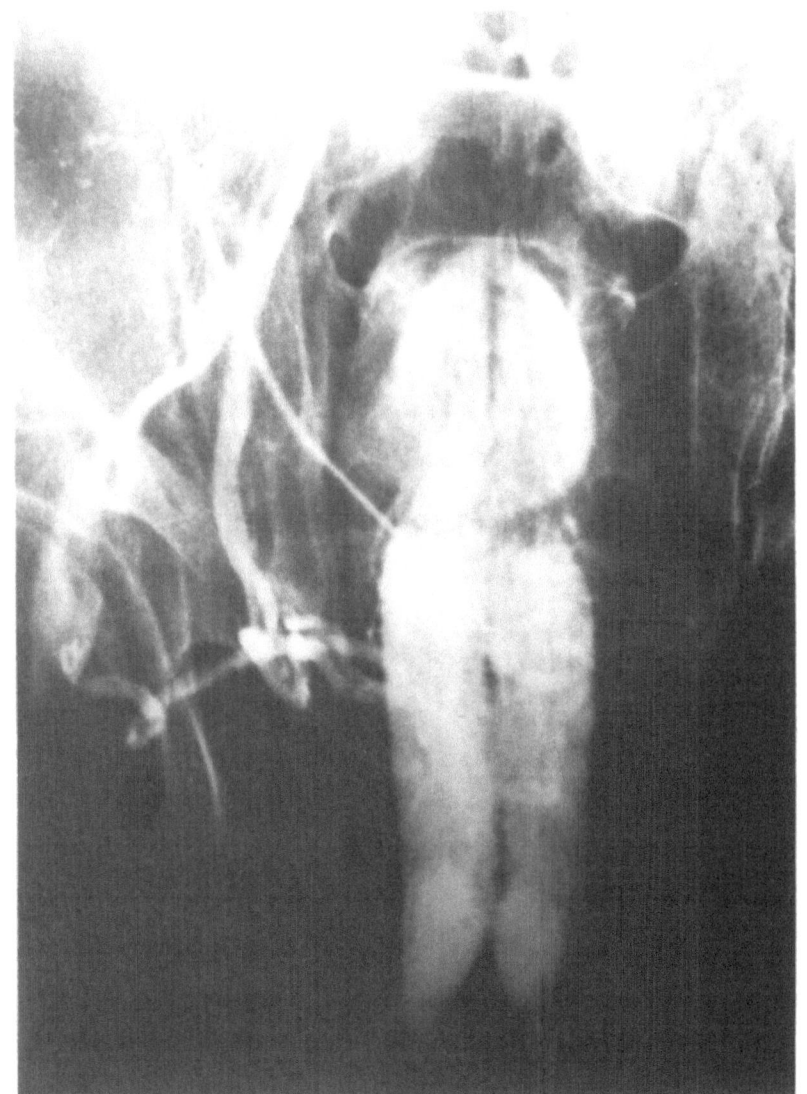

2

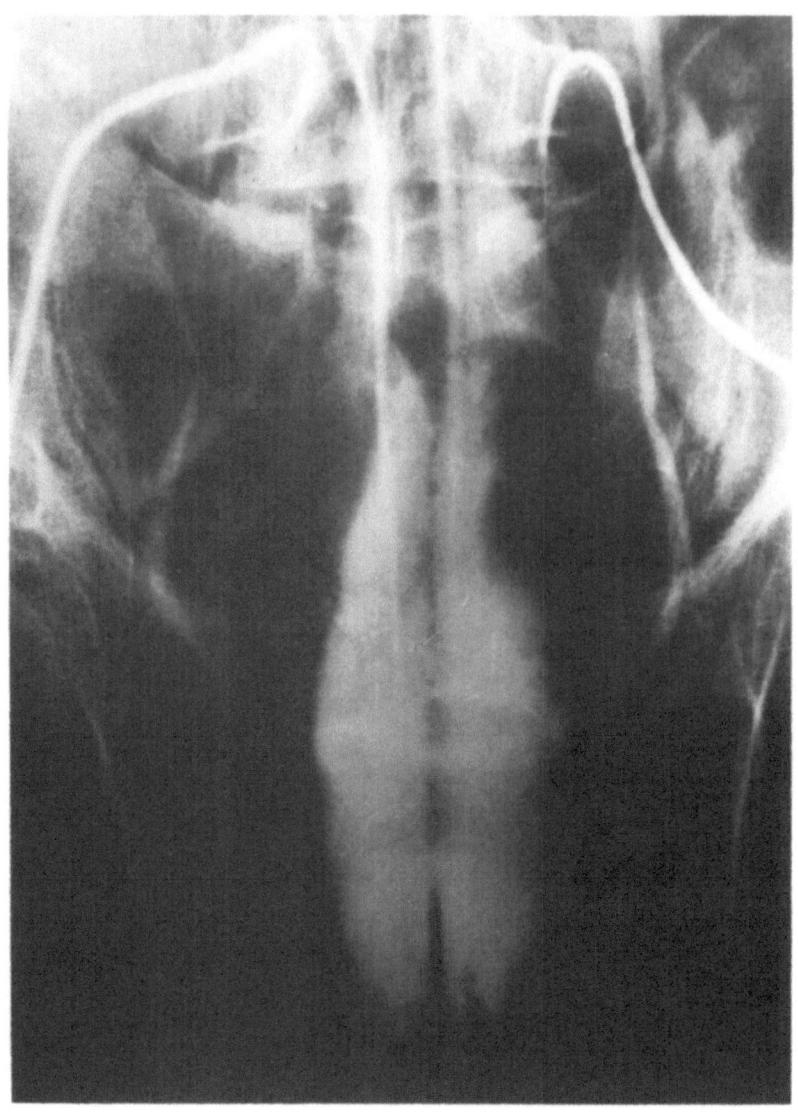

Fig. 79 - Peyronie's disease - cavernography

Normal dilatation of perineal portion of corps cavernosum.

Deficiency of expansion of penial segment of the two secondary corps cavernosum to the albuginea fibrosis.

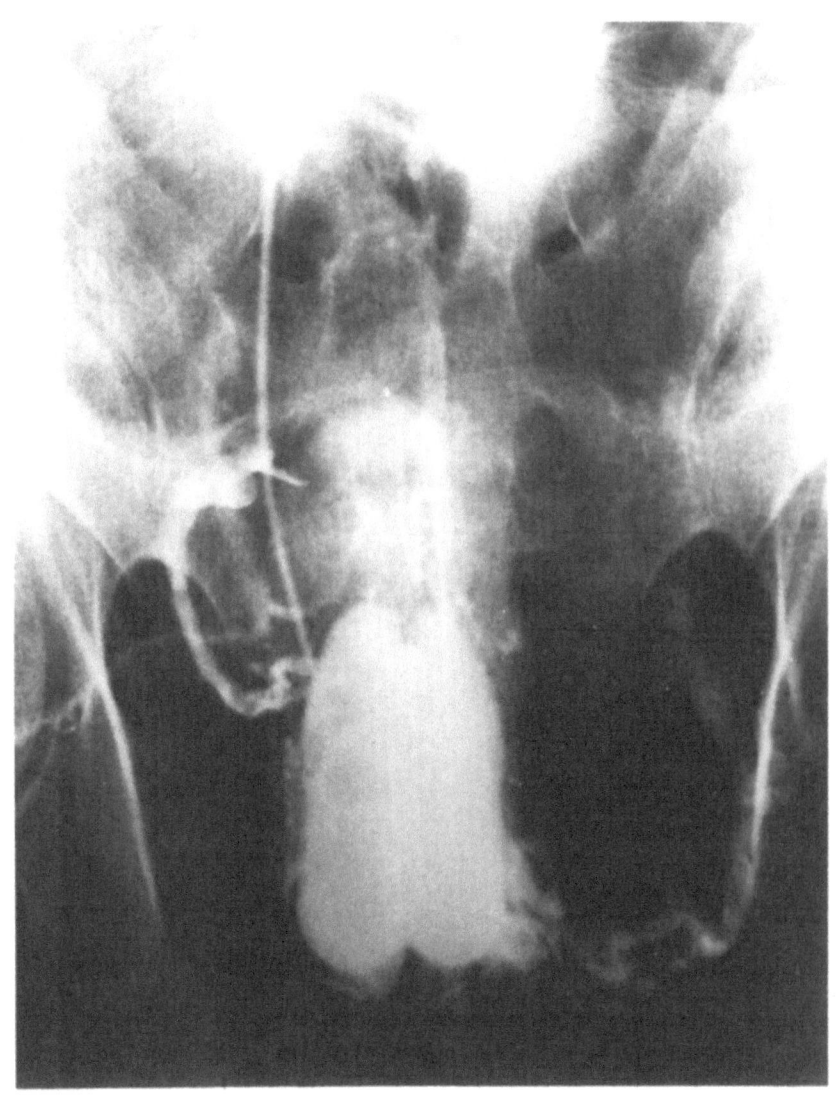

Fig. 80 - Peyronie's disease - cavernography

Atrophy of corps cavernosum, the penial portion
does not expand.

No expansion of corps cavernosum on injection.

CONCLUSION

The sexual function is a function in its own right which unjustly was confused for a long time with the function of reproduction. Among all members of the animal kingdom, man manifests the greatest discrimination between these two functions; it increases with man's degree of evolution. Sexual needs and orgasm have become drives completely distinct from the sentiment or the instinct of reproduction.

Anatomy and physiology of the sexual organs on the one hand and those of the organs of reproduction on the other hand are related but different. Impotence is substantiated organically. Its psychiatric causes are rare, contrary to conventional concepts.

It may be a symptom. It is a complication of a general disease. Therefore its treatment necessitates first that of the disease.

It may be a disease, most likely either of *neurologic* or of *vascular* nature. In the field of neurologic diseases our research has not as yet yielded any substantial results. As to vascular diseases, with the procedures developed by the surgeon of our team, the achieved positive results have convinced us of the importance to diagnose the lesion of the internal pudendal artery and the deep artery of the penis.

According to our statistics, one out of four patients has impotence of vascular origin. It would be inexcusable not to offer such a patient a chance of cure. This is what led us to the present publication.

IRRADIATION

A frequent criticism of these techniques is the excessive radiation dose to the gonads during the examinations.

This is however not the real problem, for two reasons:

1. Although it is not possible to determine precisely the amount of radiation absorbed — since this depends upon the weight of the patient, the type of screen used and the film selected by the radiologist — it can be stated that it is limited.

With experience, every serial examination can be restricted to 6-8 radiographs. Thus one selective bilateral arteriographic examination can be compared with two intravenous urographic examinations, one cavernography with one intravenous urography.

2. For these impotent patients, irradiation of the gonads is of secondary significance. It is much more important to find a therapeutic solution that will enable them to have a normal sexual relationship once again.